Natural First Aid

- **Herbal Treatments for Ailments & Injuries**

- **Emergency Preparedness**

- **Wilderness Safety**

Brigitte Mars, Herbalist AHG

CC3261042946 0544

12⁹⁵ Aw
11/99

STOREY BOOKS
Schoolhouse Road
Pownal, Vermont 05261

The mission of Storey Communications is to serve our customers by publishing practical information that encourages personal independence in harmony with the environment.

This book is intended to educate and expand one's concepts of how to deal with a crisis. It is not intended to take the place of courses in first aid or to replace medical care when needed.

Edited by Deborah Balmuth and Nancy Ringer
Cover design by Meredith Maker
Cover art production and text design by Betty Kodela
Text production by Susan Bernier
Illustrations by Alison Kolesar, except on pages iv, vi, 1, 3, and 20 by Sarah Brill; pages 93 and 117 by Beverly Duncan; page 128 by Mallory Lake; and page 131 by Charles Joslin
Indexed by Susan Olason, Indexes & Knowledge Maps
Professional assistance by Roseanna Rich

Printed in the United States by R.R. Donnelley
10 9 8 7 6 5 4 3 2 1

Library of Congress Cataloging-in-Publication Data

Mars, Brigitte.
    Natural first aid / Brigitte Mars.
      p. cm. — (A medicinal herb guide)
    Includes index.
    ISBN 1-58017-147-8 (pbk. : alk. paper)
    1. First aid in illness and injury Handbooks, manuals, etc.   2. Herbs — Therapeutic use Handbooks, manuals, etc.   3. Naturopathy Handbooks, manuals, etc.   I. Title.   II. Series.
    RC86.8 .M3875 1999
    616.02'52—dc21   99-32307
                                                           CIP

EMERGENCY NUMBERS

Fire _____

Gas Company/Public Service _____

Phone Company _____ _

Police _____

Poison Control _____

Your Address and Phone Number

_____

_____

_____

_____

Dedicated to my parents,
Rita and Morton Smookler

CONTENTS

Acknowledgments vi

Introduction 1

1 First-Aid Techniques Everyone Should
  Know: A Step-by-Step Illustrated Guide 3
    CPR 3
    The Heimlich Maneuver 11
    Bandaging Limbs 16
    Immobilization: Applying Splints and Slings 16
    The Recovery Position 18
    Moving the Injured 18
    Using Homeopathic Medicines 19

2 An A–Z Guide to Ailments and Injuries 20

3 Surviving Nature's Challenges:
  Tips and Techniques for Emergencies 93

4 Stocking a First-Aid Kit 117

5 How to Make and Use Herbal Medicines 128

Index 132

 acknowledgments

ACKNOWLEDGMENTS

A special thank you to Dr. Charles Tawa of Boulder Family Practice for his extensive knowledge of emergency medical and health care; Lorene Wapotich, herbalist, for her expertise as a wilderness emergency technician; Flame Dineen, registered midwife, for sharing her expertise; and Matthew Becker, herbalist extraordinaire.

INTRODUCTION

Stay calm. Move quickly. Know what to do. Those three rules are the foundation of natural first aid. They can mean the difference between life and death, injury and disability, a night in the hospital and a life in a nursing home.

Unfortunately, even though most of us can generally manage to stay calm and move fast during a crisis, few of us really know what to do in an emergency or when an accident occurs. Even fewer know when and how to use the herbs and other home remedies that can heal.

That's why this book was written. It contains all the techniques you need to render emergency first aid, specific instructions for over 75 injuries and conditions, and clear indications for when medical help is needed. There is also a complete list of the ingredients you'll need to stock three different first-aid kits: an herbal kit to stay at home, a survival kit to keep in your car, and a traveling kit to tuck in your handbag or briefcase as you go about your life.

With this book, you'll always be prepared. Memorize its lifesaving techniques. Learn its commonsense healing. Then supplement this knowledge by taking a first-aid and CPR course at your local Red Cross. And remember: This book is intended not as a replacement for competent medical care when it is needed, but as a guide for appropriate action *until* help can be obtained.

1

In an emergency, call for help as soon as possible. Ask the injured person if he or she has any allergies, is on any medication, or suffers from any medical conditions so that you can relay this information to medical personnel should the victim lose consciousness. If the victim is unconscious, check for medical alert bracelets. Never give food or water to an unconscious person as they may choke. And never move a person with serious injuries, especially those affecting the neck or spine. Your efforts, well meaning though they may be, could cause serious damage.

One final note: Preventing accidents and injuries is always easier than responding to them. That's why I not only keep medicines out of children's reach and in-line skates off the stairs, but also why I often visualize surrounding myself and my loved ones with an aura of light as we go off into the busy world. It's a form of prayer and my way of acknowledging and asking for divine protection. I firmly believe it has helped save my family from danger — and I urge you to use it, too.

Many blessings!

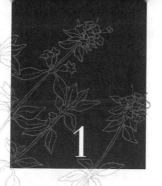

FIRST-AID TECHNIQUES EVERYONE SHOULD KNOW:
A Step-by-Step Illustrated Guide

While learning first aid might seem a daunting task, there are really only a handful of simple techniques that everyone should be familiar with. These techniques form the basis of almost all first-aid treatments and will prove invaluable if you're someday faced with an emergency situation. Although a book is a good place to start, it's always best to get instruction from a qualified health care provider before trying any of these techniques. In addition, always remember the the most important rule of medicine: First, do no harm.

The following sections on CPR and the Heimlich maneuver come straight from the American Heart Association (AHA). I strongly recommend that you contact your local chapter of the AHA to find out more about training and certification in these lifesaving techniques in your area.

CARDIOPULMONARY RESUSCITATION (CPR)

CPR is performed when someone's breathing or pulse (or both) stops. When both stop, sudden death has occurred. Sudden death has many possible causes — poisoning, drowning, choking, suffocation, electrocution, smoke inhalation — but the most common is heart attack.

Everyone should know the signals of heart attack and the actions for survival. They should also have a plan for emergency action.

Warning Signs

The warning signs of a heart attack are:
- Uncomfortable pressure, fullness, squeezing, or pain in the center of the chest that lasts more than a few minutes.
- Pain spreading to the shoulders, neck, or arms.
- Chest discomfort with lightheadedness, fainting, sweating, nausea, or shortness of breath.

Not all these signs occur in every heart attack. If some start to occur, don't wait. Get help fast.

Actions for Survival

- Recognize the signals.
- Stop whatever you're doing and sit or lie down.
- If the signals last more than a few minutes, call the local emergency number. (Usually it's 911.) If that's not possible, take the victim to the nearest hospital emergency room with emergency cardiac care.

Since incorrect chest compressions can cause internal injuries, CPR should be performed only by someone who has taken a professional course. CPR requires training, practice, and skill. This information is presented for the purpose of review for one who is trained. Keep in mind that anyone who performs CPR should pull on a pair of latex gloves if they're available.

To determine if a person is breathing, place your ear against their mouth or nose: Can you hear them exhale? Place your head or hand on their chest: Does the chest rise and fall?

> **Caution**
>
> Never practice CPR on a healthy person — it can be harmful.

Seek immediate medical attention if:
- the victim is not breathing
- breathing is noisy
- froth appears around the lips or nose
- a bluish color appears around the lips and ears

The ABC's of CPR

CPR is a procedure that's as simple as **A**irway, **B**reathing, and **C**irculation. First, assess the victim. Try to get a response from the person. Shake them gently, while calling, "Are you okay?" If the person isn't responsive, activate the emergency medical system (911 or local number). Then begin the ABC's: Airway, Breathing, and Circulation. Continue CPR without stopping until advanced life support is available.

A irway

To open the airway, gently lift the chin with one hand while pushing down on the forehead with your other hand. You want to tilt the head back. Once the airway is open, lean over and put your ear close to the victim's mouth.

- Look at the chest for movement.
- Listen for the sound of breathing.
- Feel for breath on your cheek.

If the victim is breathing, roll the person onto his or her side as a unit (the recovery position — see page 18). If none of these signs is present, the person isn't breathing. If opening the airway doesn't cause the person to sponta- neously start breathing, you'll have to provide rescue breathing.

> ### Assessment and Activation
>
> If you find an adult who has collapsed, find out if he or she is unresponsive by gently shaking a shoulder and shouting "Are you all right?" If the person doesn't respond, shout for help. If a helper is avail- able, send that person to call your emergency medical service (911 or other local number). If no help is avail- able, make the call yourself.

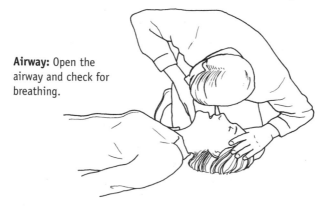

Airway: Open the airway and check for breathing.

*B*reathing

The best way to give rescue breathing is by using the mouth-to-mouth technique:

1. Using the thumb and forefinger of your hand that's on the victim's forehead, pinch the person's nose shut. Be sure to keep the heel of your hand in place so the person's head remains tilted. Keep your other hand under the person's chin, lifting up.

2. As you keep an air-tight seal with your mouth on the victim's mouth, immediately give two full breaths.

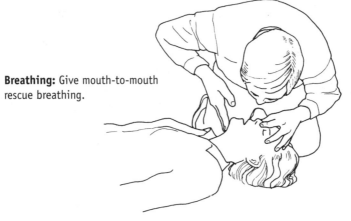

Breathing: Give mouth-to-mouth rescue breathing.

*C*irculation

After giving two full breaths, find the person's carotid artery pulse to see if the heart is still beating. To find the carotid artery pulse, take your hand that's lifting the chin and find the person's Adam's apple (voice box). Slide the tips of your fingers down the groove beside the Adam's apple and feel for the pulse.

If you can't find the pulse, in addition to rescue breathing, you'll have to provide artificial circulation.

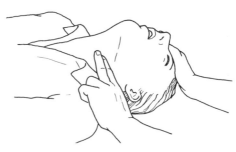

Circulation: Check for signs of a pulse.

External Chest Compression

External chest compressions provide artificial circulation. When you apply rhythmic pressure on the lower half of the victim's breastbone, you force the heart to pump blood.

To do external chest compression properly, kneel beside the victim's chest. With the middle and index fingers of your hand nearest the person's legs, find the notch where the bottom rims of the two halves of the rib cages meet in the middle of the chest. Now put the heel of one hand on the sternum (breastbone) next to the fingers that found the notch. Put your other hand on top of the hand that's in position. Be sure to keep your fingers up off the chest wall. It may be easier to do this if you interlock your fingers.

Bring your shoulders directly over the victim's sternum and press down, keeping your arms straight. If the victim is an adult, depress the sternum about 1½ to 2 inches (3.8 to 5 cm). Then completely relax the pressure on the sternum. Don't remove your hands from the victim's sternum, but do let the chest rise to its normal position between compressions. Relaxation and compression should take equal amounts of time.

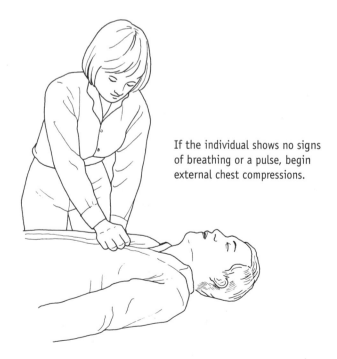

If the individual shows no signs of breathing or a pulse, begin external chest compressions.

If you must give both rescue breathing and external chest compressions, the proper rate is 15 chest compressions to 2 breaths. You must compress at a rate of 80 to 100 times per minute.

If You Suspect a Neck Injury

If you suspect that the victim may have a neck injury (such as might occur in a diving or automobile accident, for example), you must open the airway differently, using a chin-lift without tilting the head. If the airway stays blocked, tilt the head slowly and gently until the airway is open.

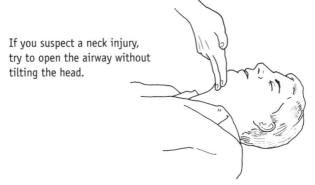

If you suspect a neck injury, try to open the airway without tilting the head.

CPR for Infants and Children

Cardiopulmonary resuscitation for infants (birth to 1 year) and children (1 to 8 years) is similar to that for adults, but there are a few important differences. They're given below.

A irway

Be careful when handling an infant. Don't tilt the head back too far. An infant's neck bends so easily that if the head is tilted back too far, the breathing passages may be blocked instead of opened.

B reathing

If an infant isn't breathing, don't try to pinch the nose shut. Cover both the mouth and nose with your mouth and breathe slowly (1.0 to 1.5 seconds per breath). Use enough volume and pressure to make the chest rise.

With a small child, pinch the nose, cover the mouth, and breathe the same as for an infant.

Text on CPR © American Heart Association. Reproduced with permission.
American Heart Association World Wide Web, 1999: www.americanheart.org.

Circulation

Check pulse. In an infant, check for a pulse by feeling on the inside of the upper arm midway between the elbow and the shoulder. Check for the pulse in a small child the same way you would in an adult.

Chest compressions. In infants and small children, use only one hand for compression. You can slip your other hand under the back of an infant to give firm support.

For infants, use only the tips of the middle and ring fingers to compress the chest at the sternum. A summary of information is given in the table below. Depress the sternum between ½ to 1 inch at a rate of at least 100 times a minute.

For small children, use only the heel of one hand (see table for position). Depress the sternum between 1 and 1½ inches, depending on the child's size. The rate should be 80 to 100 times a minute.

In the case of both infants and small children, give breaths during a pause after every fifth chest compression.

CPR for children over 8 years old is the same as for adults.

Assessment and Activation
If you don't get a response from an infant or child, send someone to call your local emergency medical service (usually 911) and begin CPR. If you're alone, do one minute of CPR before leaving to call 911. Return to the victim and continue CPR until help (EMS) arrives.

CPR FOR CHILDREN				
AGE	PART OF HAND	HAND POSITION	DEPRESS STERNUM	RATE OF COMPRESSION
Infant (birth to 1 year)	Tips of middle and ring fingers	One finger's width below line between nipples (be sure not to depress the tip of the sternum)	½ to 1 inch (1.3 to 2.5 cm)	5 compressions to 1 full breath; at least 100 compressions per minute
Child (1 to 8 years)	Heel of hand	Sternum (same as adults)	1 to 1½ inches (2.5 to 3.8 cm)	5 compressions to 1 full breath; 80 to 100 compressions per minute

Text on CPR © American Heart Association. Reproduced with permission. American Heart Association World Wide Web, 1999: www.americanheart.org.

Remember

A irway: Is the victim unresponsive? If so, shout for help, position the child, and open the airway.

B reathing: Check for breathing. If there's no breathing, give 2 full breaths. Look for chest rise, listen for sounds of breathing, feel for breath on your cheek

C irculation: If the victim still isn't breathing, attempt to check the carotid pulse for a few seconds. If there's no pulse or you can't locate the pulse and the child is still unresponsive, begin 1 minute of CPR. Then leave to activate the local EMS system or send someone else to activate the local emergency number while you perform CPR. Continue to do CPR until help (EMS) arrives.

Alternate compressions and rescue breathing at the proper ratio.
- For adults and children over 8 years old the ratio is 15 compressions to 2 full breaths at a rate of 80 to 100 compressions per minute.
- For children 1 to 8 years old the proper ratio is 5 compressions to 1 full breath at a rate of 80 to 100 compressions per minute.
- For infants the proper ratio is 5 compressions to 1 full breath at a rate of at least 100 compressions per minute.

Periodic practice in CPR is essential to keep your skills at the level they need to be. Someone's life may depend on how well you remember — and apply — the steps in CPR. Have your CPR skills and knowledge tested at least once a year. It could enable you to save a life.

Waiting for Help

If an individual doesn't regain consciousness, keep CPR going for at least an hour whether it's a child or an adult. In a group, take turns. Don't stop until medical help arrives.

THE HEIMLICH MANEUVER

The Heimlich maneuver is used to aid an individual who is choking. In effect, the under-the-diaphragm series of thrusts forces enough air from the lungs to artificially create a cough, which is intended to move or expel a foreign object that is obstructing the victim's breathing. After performing the Heimlich maneuver, have the victim examined by a medical professional.

The technique should only be performed when the victim's airway is completely obstructed by a foreign object. The Heimlich maneuver is *not* recommended if he or she can cough or speak. So before beginning, encourage the person who is choking to cough. Besides, this may be enough to dislodge any blockage.

If the victim is having trouble coughing or breathing, however, ask if he is choking:

- **If he can cough or speak,** let him try to expel the blockage on his own.
- **If he can't cough but is breathing,** his airway is only partially obstructed. Arrange for immediate transport to an emergency medical facility to remove the blockage.
- **If he cannot speak or cough,** his airway is obstructed. Get someone to call for medical help while you perform the lifesaving Heimlich maneuver.

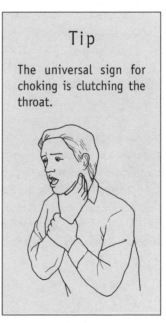

Tip

The universal sign for choking is clutching the throat.

An Illustrated Guide to the Heimlich Maneuver

If the victim is conscious:

1. Ask, "Are you choking?" If the victim can speak, cough, or breathe, do not interfere.

Text on Heimlich maneuver © American Heart Association. Reproduced with permission.
American Heart Association World Wide Web, 1999: www.americanheart.org.

2. If the victim cannot speak, cough, or breathe, give abdominal thrusts (the Heimlich maneuver) until the foreign object is expelled or the victim becomes unconscious.

Note: If the victim is extremely obese or in the late stages of pregnancy, give chest thrusts.

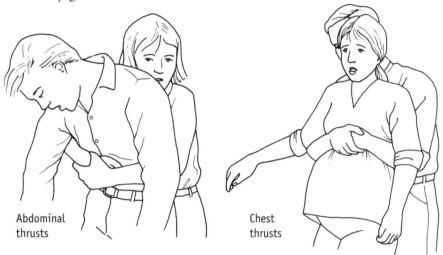

Abdominal thrusts

Chest thrusts

3. Be persistent. Continue uninterrupted until the obstruction is relieved or advanced life support is available. In either case the victim should be examined by a physician as soon as possible.

If the victim becomes unconscious:

4. Activate the emergency medical system (911 or local number).

5. Perform a tongue-jaw lift followed by a finger sweep to try to remove the foreign object.

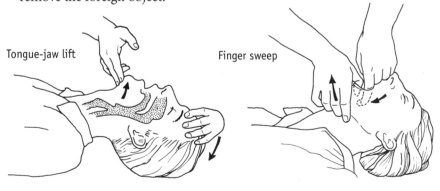

Tongue-jaw lift

Finger sweep

6. Open the airway and try to give 2 slow rescue breaths. If unsuccessful, reposition the head and try again.

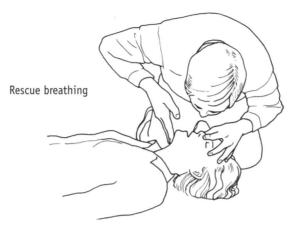

Rescue breathing

7. If unsuccessful, give up to 5 abdominal thrusts (the Heimlich maneuver).

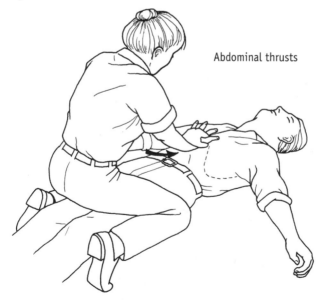

Abdominal thrusts

8. Repeat steps 5 through 7 until effective. If the victim resumes effective breathing, place in the recovery position.

Text on Heimlich maneuver © American Heart Association. Reproduced with permission.
American Heart Association World Wide Web, 1999: www.americanheart.org.

9. After the obstruction is removed, begin the ABC's of CPR if necessary (see page 5).

10. Be persistent. Continue uninterrupted until the obstruction is relieved or advanced life support is available. When successful, have the victim examined by a physician as soon as possible.

The Heimlich Maneuver for Infants and Children

When there are signs of choking in an infant (birth to 1 year) or child (1 to 8 years):

- If the infant or child is breathing and continues to be able to speak or cough, do not interfere, but take to an advanced life support facility.
- If the infant or child has a fever or history of illness, the air passages may be swollen. Take to an emergency care facility.
- If the infant or child has ineffective coughing and high-pitched inspirations and is unable to speak or cry, then immediately begin the obstructed airway sequence described below.

If an infant is conscious:

1. Support the infant's head and neck with one hand firmly holding the jaw. Place the infant face-down on your forearm, keeping the head lower than the trunk.

2. With the heel of your free hand, deliver up to 5 back blows forcefully between the infant's shoulder blades.

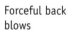
Forceful back blows

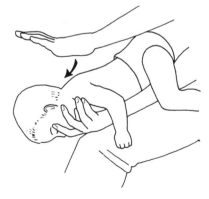

3. Supporting the head, sandwich the infant between your hands and arms and turn the infant on his or her back, keeping the head lower than the trunk. Using two fingers, deliver up to 5 thrusts over the lower half of the breastbone (sternum).

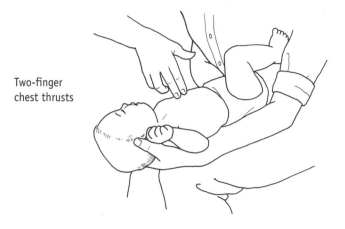

Two-finger
chest thrusts

If the infant becomes unconscious:
1. Call for help. If someone comes, that person should activate the emergency medical system (911 or local number).
2. Open the airway (head tilt and chin lift) and try to give 2 slow rescue breaths. If the airway is still obstructed, reposition the head and try again to give rescue breaths.
3. Give up to 5 back blows, then up to 5 chest thrusts.
4. Perform a tongue-jaw lift, and if you see the obstructing object, perform a finger sweep to remove it.
5. If the foreign body is not removed, repeat steps 2 through 4 until successful. If the infant resumes effective breathing, place in the recovery position.
6. If the airway obstruction is not relieved after 1 minute, activate the emergency medical system (usually 911).
7. If the foreign body is removed and the victim is not breathing, begin the ABC's of CPR for infants.

8. When successful, have the infant examined by a health-care professional as soon as possible.

If a child is conscious, perform the Heimlich maneuver as described for adults.

If the child becomes unconscious:
Continue as for an adult, but do not perform blind finger sweeps. Instead, perform a tongue-jaw lift and try to remove the foreign object only if you see it.

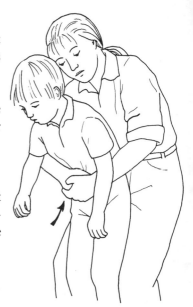

BANDAGING LIMBS

Bandages should be long enough to encircle the limb, and at least an inch wider than the wound. Keep them loose enough to avoid impairing circulation, and bandage a limb in the position in which it will remain during the transport or while the wound heals.

  1. Begin by placing the end of the bandage on the limb.

  2. Make a firm turn around the limb to hold the bandage's end in place. Secure the bandage with first-aid tape, a safety pin, or by cutting the end of the bandage in two, putting one end on each side of the limb, and then tying the ends into a knot.

IMMOBILIZATION: APPLYING SPLINTS AND SLINGS

Splints are support devices used to immobilize a potentially fractured bone or injured joint when medical attention is not immediately available. Slings are used to immobilize the splinted limb. Unless you are in a situation where medical attention is unavailable, they should only be applied by those who are trained to do so. However, if you are the only one available in an emergency situation, here are the basics.

A splint can be fashioned from rolled-up newspapers, rolled blankets, pillows, boards, and so forth. Ideally, a splint should be long enough to extend past either end of a suspected fracture and past the nearest joints. It is important to splint an injury in the position you found it. Do not attempt to move or straighten an injured limb.

To hold a splint in place, use bandannas, neckties, or strips of cloth as a sling. Tie the splint above and below the injury. Secure the joints above and below the injury. The splint should provide firm support for the injury while allowing for good circulation. Indications that circulation is impeded include blue or pale fingers or toes on the splinted limb. Have all the knots on the same side, and do not allow them to press into the injury. Here's how to apply splints and/or slings on specific areas:

Wrist or lower arm: Put the injured arm across the patient's torso with the elbow at a right angle. The palm should be in, the thumb up. Splint each side of the arm from the elbow to beyond the wrist, leaving the fingers visible. Check the fingers frequently to see if circulation is impeded by tight bandages.

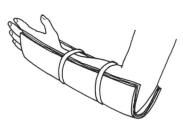
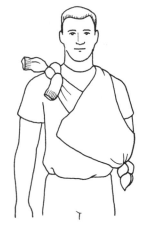

In emergency situations, splints and slings can be improvised. In this case, rolled sturdy paper or cardboard makes an adequate splint, and a long-sleeved shirt has been tied as a sling.

Finger and toe: Tape the injured finger or toe to the one next to it with cotton or other soft material between the two.

Foot and ankle: Remove the shoe from the injured appendage. Tie padding, such as towels, blankets, or spare clothing, around the shin and foot, leaving the toes exposed. Check the toes frequently to see that circulation is not impeded by tight bandages.

THE RECOVERY POSITION

The recovery position prevents the windpipe from getting blocked by saliva, blood, or the tongue. *Never place a person with a suspected spinal injury into the recovery position.* For all others, here's what to do:

1. Place the injured person flat on the ground on his or her stomach. Turn his or her head to the side, tilting it back to open the airway. Loosen any constrictive clothing. Lay the arm that the head is turned away from along the patient's side, keeping it straight. Place the other arm across the chest, and the ankle on that same side over the other ankle.

2. Straighten the injured person's throat by tilting his head back to allow for free breathing. Bend the upper arm toward the head. Bend the upper leg to prop the lower body.

If the patient is too heavy for you to move, have another person support the head while you turn the body with both hands.

If the individual has a broken leg or arm, lay them in the recovery position with a rolled blanket under the uninjured side.

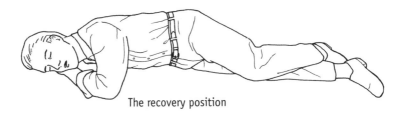

The recovery position

MOVING THE INJURED

Never move a person with serious injuries, especially if you suspect a neck or spinal injury. For all others, here's what to do:

1. Immobilize any injured parts before moving.

2. If the injured person is unable to walk, he or she can be dragged on a blanket or coat if necessary — lengthwise rather than sideways, and carefully secured so that he or she doesn't roll off the blanket during transport. Place a pillow under the head and neck of an unconscious victim to avoid inadvertently closing his or her airway.

3. If the injured individual is conscious, sitting up, does not have a leg injury, but is unable to walk, two people can clasp hands to make a chair.

USING HOMEOPATHIC MEDICINES

Homeopathy is a system of medicine based on the principle that "like cures like." For example, the remedy suggested for treating poison ivy rashes is *Rhus tox,* which is made from the poison ivy plant itself. In large amounts, some of the ingredients in homeopathic remedies can be toxic. However, the preparations are so diluted that what you are getting is the "energy" of the remedy that can help stimulate the body's own healing process.

Homeopathic Dosages

Homeopathic remedies are usually taken by placing 4 pellets under the tongue every 4 hours for the first few days following an injury or onset of an illness, or until results are seen. Children should take smaller doses:

Infants under 1 year of age	1 pellet every 4 hours
Children ages 1 to 5 years	2 pellets every 4 hours
Children ages 6 to 12 years	3 pellets every 4 hours
Children over 12 years of age	Adult dosage

In all cases, consult with a trained practitioner before treating children with homeopathy. And remember, homeopathic medicines use minute doses of sometimes toxic substances that can be dangerous in large amounts — stick with the homeopathic dose.

RESCUE REMEDY FOR EMERGENCIES

Rescue Remedy is a homeopathic preparation (available in health food stores) made from five flower essences. It can be given for trauma, accidents, and emotional distress to help restore calm and bolster confidence. The essences in the mixture are: Star of Bethlehem for shock, Rock Rose for terror and panic, Impatiens for stress and tension, Cherry Plum for despair and fear of losing control, and Clematis for loss of consciousness or feeling "out of it." Two to four drops can be placed under the tongue and held there a minute or so before swallowing. The drops can also be mixed into a small glass of water and sipped. If the person to whom you are administering first aid is unconscious, place the drops on the lips, wrists, back of the neck, or behind the ears.

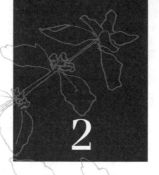

2

AN A–Z GUIDE TO
AILMENTS AND INJURIES

ABDOMINAL INJURIES (See also *Bruises* or *Stomach Pain*)

Seek immediate medical attention if the injured individual experiences:

- Heavy bleeding
- Nausea or vomiting
- Muscle spasms
- Faintness
- Tenderness or pain
- Discoloration of urine, stool, vomit, or sputum
- Swelling

While you wait for medical attention:

1. Keep the injured person as comfortable and still as possible. Loosen tight clothes at neck and waist, then cover the injured person with a blanket. If you suspect internal injuries, do not move the individual. If he or she is bleeding from an abdominal wound, however, position them as follows (after slipping on a pair of latex gloves, if possible):

- *If the wound is lengthwise to the body,* place the injured person on his or her back, with the feet slightly elevated. Do not raise the head as it will tense abdominal muscles that affect the wound.

- *If the wound is across the abdomen,* have the individual lay on his or her back, but place a pillow or a clean folded cloth behind the head and knees. This will relax the abdominal muscles and help keep the wound closed.

- *If bleeding, try to keep the injured area clean.* Gently remove the clothing surrounding the injury. If any internal parts are protruding, do not push them back inside. Place a dressing or folded clean cloth on the wound and bind it loosely in place with tape or a bandage. Do not press down on the bandage.

2. Do not allow the injured person to eat or drink. If he or she asks for a drink, dip a cloth in water and moisten the lips. Two drops of Rescue Remedy can be added to 8 ounces (230 ml) of water and the cloth dipped in that solution, if desired.

ABRASIONS AND LACERATIONS (See also *Shock*)

A superficial cut is called an abrasion. A deep cut is called a laceration.

Seek immediate medical attention if the wound:

- Is spurting blood
- Is so wide you suspect the wound will require stitches
- Looks deep
- Affects a finger or joint
- Is due to a broken bone
- Is due to a human or animal bite
- Was caused by a rusty, dirty object that may carry the tetanus toxin
- Was caused by an object that is still embedded
- Was caused by a knife or other sharp object

Protect Yourself

Whenever you are dealing with open wounds, wear latex gloves or use some other form of barrier to protect yourself against blood-borne pathogens, such as the HIV virus and hepatitis.

While you wait for medical attention:

1. Unless you suspect a fracture, raise the wounded area above the heart to help reduce bleeding.

2. Apply pressure to the wound. Slip on a pair of latex gloves if you have them. As long as nothing's embedded in a bleeding wound, cover it with the cleanest cloth available and apply direct pressure. If the cloth gets soaked through, add more cloths and continue to press firmly. Do not remove any of the cloths. If no cloth is available, use your hand or fingers. Maintain continuous pressure until the bleeding has ceased. Reapply if necessary.

3. Try to keep the person calm. Stress can elevate blood pressure and thus increase blood loss.

4. Apply pressure to the main arteries. If bleeding continues, press on the appropriate point as indicated in the illustrations below. Stop pressing once bleeding has stopped.

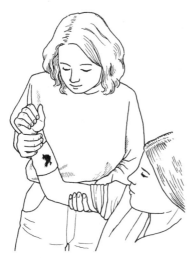

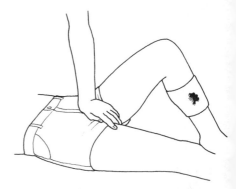

To stop bleeding in the arm, hold the limb up at a right angle to the body. Grasp the arm firmly with the thumb on the outside and the remaining fingers firmly on the inside of the upper arm, over the brachial artery.

To stop bleeding in the legs, have the injured person lie flat on his or her back. Press the heel of your hand on the femoral artery as it crosses the crease between thigh and groin.

At-Home First Aid for Abrasions and Lacerations

If the wound does not require immediate medical care, your job is to clean it, stop the bleeding, and set the stage for healing. Here's how:

1. Clean the wound. Wash your hands and the injured area with soap and water, then rinse with running water. Blot dry. Because bleeding allows the wound to clean itself, encourage the wound to bleed just a bit by gently pressing around the injured area. If there is visible dirt in the wound, use sterile gauze to wipe the dirt out. Do not use cotton balls, as they can leave little fibers in the wound.

When the wound is clean, there are several household, herbal, and homeopathic remedies you can have ready in an instant to reduce blood flow. They're listed below.

2. Apply a bandage. If the wound is large or going to be exposed to dust and dirt, apply sterile gauze, and secure with adhesive tape.

If you're in an area in which plantain grows, you can pick some leaves, wash and shred them, then mix with warm water until well saturated. Apply topically as a poultice under the bandage (or instead of a bandage, if one is unavailable).

Household remedies.

Cayenne powder. Applied topically, it stings but does indeed encourage wounds to stop bleeding.

Spider webs. Believe it or not, spider webs contain a coagulating substance that can be applied to cuts. Just make sure the spider has left the web!

Herbal remedies.

Herbal salves. Any herbal salve containing infection-fighting herbs such as echinacea, calendula, goldenseal, chaparral, osha, or lavender, or bee propolis or tea tree essential oil may also aid healing.

Cranesbill, shepherd's purse, tienchi ginseng *(Panax pseudo-ginseng),* and yarrow. Use any of these as a tincture, powdered in a blend, or crushed and applied as a poultice. (See instructions for making a tincture or poultice in chapter 5.)

Homeopathic remedies. Depending on the situation described, take 4 pellets (dissolved under the tongue) of one of the following to help reduce bleeding:

Aconitum for severe bleeding, especially if the person is going into shock and exhibits anxiety and fear

Hypericum for wounds in which there are lots of nerve endings — fingertips, for example — and for wounds in which the injured person feels a sharp, shooting pain

Ledum for deep puncture wounds, especially if the area is swollen, reddish, and numb or cold

Phosphorus for small wounds that bleed heavily

Veratrum album for victims who are bleeding and on the verge of shock

Follow-Up Care for Abrasions and Lacerations

Echinacea tincture can be taken orally to help prevent infection; gotu kola tincture can promote connective tissue repair. Take 1 dropperful 4 times daily for 7 to 10 days.

ALCOHOL POISONING (See also *Drug/Alcohol Overdose*)

Seek immediate medical attention if the individual:

- Cannot be roused
- Has diabetes
- Has a slow pulse
- Is having difficulty breathing
- Has dilated pupils
- Has pale skin or is sweating
- Cannot stop vomiting

While you wait for medical attention, loosen any tight or restrictive clothing. If the individual is unconscious, place them in the recovery position. Monitor breathing; if the individual stops breathing, initiate CPR.

ALLERGIC REACTION (acute) (See also *Hives*)

Seek immediate medical attention if the individual:
- Has difficulty breathing
- Becomes weak
- Experiences nausea
- Develops facial swelling

While you wait for medical attention:

1. Think. Ask the victim if he or she has any known allergies. Do your best to figure out what caused the allergic reaction. Prevent further ingestion or contact.

2. Reach for ephedra. If breathing is impaired give 2 dropperfuls of ephedra tincture to dilate bronchioles and prevent anaphylactic shock. In emergencies of severe allergies, take in addition a dose of 1 teaspoon (5 ml) baking soda mixed in a glass of water to alleviate symptoms. *Caution:* Ephedra should not be used by those taking medication for heart conditions or high blood pressure. Ephedra should be used with caution by those suffering from angina, diabetes, glaucoma, heart disease, high blood pressure, enlarged prostate gland, or overactive thyroid gland — do not exceed the recommended dosage!

ANIMAL BITES AND SCRATCHES

Seek immediate medical attention if the bite:
- Was inflicted by a human or wild animal
- Is on the face
- Happens to a child who has allergic tendencies
- Shows signs of infection, such as pus formation or fever, or signs of nerve or blood vessel damage — a bluish discoloration

While you wait for medical attention:

1. Clean the wound. Wash the bitten or scratched area with an antiseptic soap and hot water. After washing, flush the wound by running the hot water over it for ten minutes. Because bleeding helps clean the wound, encourage the wound to bleed just a bit by gently pressing around the injured area.

2. Apply an antiseptic and dressing. Lavender or tea tree essential oil, echinacea tincture, or povidone-iodine can all be topically applied to further disinfect the wound. Cover the wound with a dry, sterile dressing, and secure with a bandage or adhesive tape.

At-Home First Aid for Animal Bites and Scratches

If the bite doesn't require emergency care, clean and disinfect the wound as noted above.

Follow-Up Care

To prevent infection, take extra vitamin C (1,000 mg 3 times daily) as well as 1 dropperful of echinacea and/or calendula tincture several times daily for 3 days after the injury occurs.

You can also prevent infection with homeopathic remedies. Take 4 pellets dissolved under the tongue 4 times daily of the following, depending on the situation:

Acetic acid for cat bites

Apis if the wound is hot and stingy and cold applications bring relief

Lachesis for dog bites

Ledum if the bite is deep, especially if the area is swollen, red, and feels cold

ANKLE INJURY (See *Sprains and Strains*)

ASTHMA ATTACKS

Seek immediate medical attention if the individual:

• Is wheezing or not getting enough oxygen
• Is showing signs of cyanosis, including bluish lips and nail beds, pale color

While you wait for medical attention:

1. Follow the doctor's instructions. Asthma attacks can be fatal, so make sure you administer any medication that was prescribed by the individual's doctor.

2. Have the individual sit up straight in a chair. Then ask him or her to lean forward and rest their forearms on a table. Elbows should be pointed away from the body.

3. Offer a beverage. Coffee, black tea, or a hot liquid like clear soup can help break up congestion and dilate the airway. If readily available, lobelia tea (see below) is also beneficial.

4. Apply a cold water compress to the chest. In some cases, it may help stop the attack.

At-Home First Aid

Asthma attacks can be fatal, so if the symptoms are not relieved by natural remedies, seek medical attention. For more mild attacks of asthma, or for wheezing or general congestion of the airway, there are several simple remedies that can be useful:

Household remedies.
  Warming spices. Ginger can help increase circulation to the lungs —
  have the individual chew on a piece of candied ginger or apply a
  towel soaked in ginger tea to the chest or back. If the person feels up
  to eating, garlicky or spicy foods can help dilate constricted airways.

Herbal remedies. Beneficial herbal teas to try include:

Fenugreek *(Trigonella foenum gracem)*. This will help break up mucus and subdue inflammation of the respiratory system.

Lobelia *(Lobelia inflata)*. Tea made from lobelia stimulates the respiratory system and helps stop lung spasms. Make the tea with one-fourth the normal amount of herbs (¼ teaspoon [1 ml] per cup [230 ml] water), or just add 5–10 drops of tincture to 1 cup (230 ml) of warm water.

Garlic. Blend a clove of garlic into 1 cup (230 ml) of hot water and sip.

Homeopathic remedies. For each of the situations described, try 4 pellets of the remedy indicated, dissolved under the tongue.

Arsenicum can help control a mild asthma attack.

Ipecac is appropriate if there is excess mucus that the patient is unable to cough up, or cough spasms that result in vomiting.

Spongia tosta can be used for loud wheezing.

Follow-Up Care and Prevention for Asthma Attacks

If you have asthma, be on the lookout for possible food allergens. Avoid food additives such as sulphur dioxide — often added to dried fruits and wine, it's a common asthma trigger — and eat lots of beta carotene–rich foods like carrots, winter squash, and sweet potatoes. Chlorophyll-rich greens such as kale and collards are good, too, because they strengthen the mucous membranes and improve oxygen metabolism. Pungent foods like garlic and onions can help open the airway. Minimize your intake of dairy and wheat products, or any products that contain yeast, as they are common allergens and can also contribute to excess phlegm.

Strengthen your respiratory system by keeping air passages clean and avoiding pollutants such as smoke, dust, inhaled chemicals, and so on.

BACK AND NECK INJURIES

Seek immediate medical assistance for any spine or neck injury. Symptoms include:
- Pain in the back
- Pain in the back of the neck
- Lack of feeling in the lower limbs

While you wait for medical attention:

1. Do not move the injured person.

2. Caution him or her to lie still.

3. Immobilize the body by carefully putting soft, solid objects (such as rocks covered with towels) against it.

4. Make a cervical support by placing a folded towel on either side of the neck.

BEE STINGS (See *Stings [Bee, Hornet, and Wasp]*)

Seek immediate medical attention if:
- The individual's tongue swells
- The individual is wheezing or has difficulty breathing
- You observe skin flushing or a sudden-onset rash
- The individual develops a severe cough
- The individual complains of blurred vision
- The individual vomits or complains of nausea

While you wait for medical attention:

1. Remove the stinger. Being careful not to squeeze the venom sac at the base of the stinger, gently pull out the stinger by dragging the edge of the fingernail or a credit card across the embedded stinger in the opposite direction from its entry. If this is ineffective, then use tweezers. Remove the stinger as quickly as possible as the venom sac can release poisons for two or three minutes.

2. Inject epinephrine, if available. If the individual is allergic (and *only* if the individual is allergic), check to see if she is carrying a special "pen" that injects epinephrine. Many people who know they are allergic to bee stings carry them. The epinephrine will help dilate the airway and prevent anaphylactic shock.

BLACK EYE (See also *Bruises*)

Seek immediate attention if:
- The eye is bleeding
- Visual disturbances persist

While you wait for medical attention, gently apply a cold compress or ice pack.

At-Home First Aid

Black eyes are a common injury that are easy to care for at home. Here are some suggestions:

Household remedies.
   Cold compress. Apply a cold compress over the closed eye to minimize swelling and reduce pain. Keep the compress in place for at least a half hour, then remove. If, after 10 minutes, pain and swelling persist, replace the cold compress. Continue this on/off cycle as necessary.

Poultice. Make a poultice from plantain or grated raw potato and place it over the closed eye.

Homeopathic remedies. For the conditions described below, take 4 pellets (dissolved under the tongue) of the suggested remedy.

Ledum is useful if cold makes the area feel better while warmth makes it feel worse.

Hypericum can help relieve excessive pain.

Arnica can help if there is injury to the soft tissue above or below the eye, or if cold water applications help relieve the pain and the injury is either above or below the eye.

Follow-Up Care for Black Eye

To alleviate irritation and inflammation, take 1 dropperful of eyebright tincture and 1 to 2 500-mg bilberry capsules 2 times daily for up to six weeks after the injury. Wear sunglasses to protect the injured eye, and seek medical attention if vision problems develop.

BLEEDING (See also *Abrasions and Lacerations* or *Nosebleeds*)

Seek immediate medical attention if:
- An object is deeply embedded in a wound *(Do not remove it!)*
- The wound is bleeding heavily
- The person becomes unconscious
- Any body part has been severed

While you wait for medical attention:

1. Unless you suspect a fracture, raise the wounded area above the heart to help reduce bleeding. If the individual is bleeding from the ears, mouth, or nose, help him or her into a semi-sitting position, then turn the head slightly toward the side from which blood is draining.

2. Apply pressure to the wound. Slip on a pair of latex gloves if you have them. Then, as long as nothing's embedded in the wound, cover it with the cleanest cloth available and apply direct pressure. If the cloth gets soaked through, add more cloths and continue to press firmly. Do not remove any of the cloths. If no cloth is available, use your hand or fingers. Maintain continuous pressure until the bleeding has ceased.

If there is an embedded object in the wound, cover the wound with a clean cloth, adding more cloths as needed. Do not apply pressure to injury site. If bleeding continues, control it by applying pressure to the main artery as described in step 4.

3. Try to keep the person calm. Stress can elevate blood pressure and thus increase blood loss.

4. Apply pressure to the main arteries. If bleeding continues, press on the appropriate point as indicated in the illustrations below. Stop pressing once bleeding has stopped.

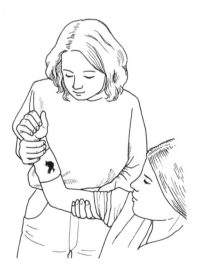

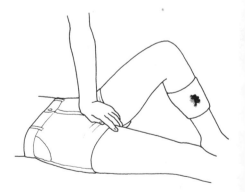

To stop bleeding in the arm, hold the limb up at a right angle to the body. Grasp the arm firmly with the thumb on the outside and the remaining fingers firmly on the inside of the upper arm, over the brachial artery.

To stop bleeding in the legs, have the injured person lie flat on his or her back. Press the heel of your hand on the femoral artery as it crosses the crease between thigh and groin.

5. If a limb has been amputated, apply a tourniquet. Wrap a strip of cloth twice around the affected limb just above the wound, tie one overhand knot, place a stick across the knot, and tie a full knot; the stick is held between these two knots. Twist the stick until the bleeding has stopped, then tie the stick in place. Note the time of application. Tourniquets must not be left on for more than 15 minutes, or you run the risk of further amputation. Release the tourniquet slowly when bleeding stops.

6. If a body part has been severed, try to keep it cold. Wrap it with a clean cloth, put it in a plastic bag, pack it in ice, and bring it with you to the medical facility.

BLISTERS

At-Home First Aid

Relieve any pressure on the blister and leave it unbroken. Then:

1. Cleanse. Wash the area gently with soap and water.

2. Disinfect. If the blister is accidentally broken, apply a few drops of lavender oil or echinacea tincture to the area.

3. Bandage. Cover with a breathable adhesive dressing.

Follow-Up Care

For both broken and unbroken blisters, apply lavender essential oil 3 times daily until the blister disappears.

BREATHING DIFFICULTIES (See also *Asthma Attacks*)

Seek immediate medical attention if:
- The individual is not breathing
- The individual's breathing is noisy
- A froth appears around the lips or nose
- A bluish color appears around the lips and ears

While you wait for medical attention:

Evaluate the need for CPR or the Heimlich maneuver. If the individual is having trouble coughing or breathing, ask if he is choking:

- **If he can cough or speak,** let him try to expel the blockage on his own.
- **If he can't cough but is breathing,** his airway is only partially obstructed. Arrange for immediate transport to an emergency medical facility to remove the blockage.
- **If he cannot speak, cough, or breathe,** his airway is obstructed. Get someone to call for medical help while you perform the lifesaving Heimlich maneuver (see page 11).

BROKEN BONES (See *Fractures*)

BRUISES

At-Home First Aid

Bruises occur when the skin is struck with such force that blood vessels break and leak, and blood fills the damaged tissues below the surface of the skin, yet the skin is unbroken. A large, deeply discolored area may indicate underlying injuries and should be examined by a health-care professional. But keep in mind that some injuries may not be immediately apparent. If pain from a bruise gets worse rather than better during the 24 hours following the injury, see a doctor. In the meantime, here's how you can help the bruise heal:

Household remedies.
　Cold packs. Ice packs or towels soaked in cold water can be used to reduce swelling. Apply for 20 minutes, then remove for 20 minutes, and repeat as necessary.

Elevation. Elevate bruised limb to minimize swelling.

Poultices. The inner skin of a fresh ripe banana, grated raw potato, grated onion, cabbage leaf, green clay mixed with apple cider vinegar, parsley, grated ginger, tofu, and wheat grass all make good poultices for bruises.

Herbal remedies.

Comfrey. A poultice made from comfrey will help relieve the pain and swelling.

Lavender. The essential oil (no more than 5 drops) can be applied directly to the bruise to encourage healing.

Homeopathic remedies. One of the most common remedies for bruising is *Arnica* — rub gently on unbroken skin to soothe deep bruises. Other homeopathic remedies to take internally (4 pellets 4 times daily, dissolved under the tongue) include:

Ruta graveolens to help relieve pain from a bruised bone; most often used when it is the elbow, kneecap, or shin that has been bruised

Hypericum for bruises to sensitive areas such as fingertips, lips, nose, or eyes

Bellis for bruising with swelling that is worse from pressure and better from active motion or rest

Ledum for bruising with extreme tenderness, when the tenderness is made better from cold and rest, worse from warmth and motion

Rhus tox when there is swelling and inflammation around soft tissue and the joint feels better after having moved a bit

Follow-Up Care for Bruises

If swelling and inflammation have subsided 24 hours after the bruise appears, begin to apply heat to stimulate healing blood flow to the area.

Prevention of Bruises

If you bruise easily, take a 1,000-mg supplement of vitamin C with bioflavonoids and rutin daily to help strengthen the capillaries. Also include plenty of leafy green vegetables and soybeans in your diet. Both are rich sources of vitamin K, a nutrient known to improve your blood's ability to clot.

Bruising easily can also indicate a nutritional deficiency, or weakness in the spleen and kidneys. Or it can be the side effect of certain medications or frequent use of nonsteroidal anti-inflammatories, such as ibuprofen. If you seem to get a lot of bruises for no apparent reason, check with your doctor.

BUG BITES (See also *Spider Bites* or *Stings [Bee, Hornet, and Wasp]*)

At-Home First Aid

Here's what to do for insect bites:

Ants. Treat ant bites topically with apple cider vinegar, green clay moistened with vinegar or water, cucumber juice, or a plantain leaf poultice. You can also try applying mud or a paste of baking soda and apple cider vinegar to help neutralize the formic acid in the bite.

Caterpillars and centipedes. When brushing off hairy caterpillars, do so from tail to head, or irritating hairs may remain in your skin. Apply lavender essential oil to their bites. Echinacea tincture can be used topically and internally (1 dropperful 3–4 times daily).

Mosquitoes. Apply mud, witch hazel, lemon juice, moistened vitamin C powder, apple cider vinegar, peppermint, a plantain leaf poultice, or lavender or tea tree essential oils to the bite.

Ticks. Brush them off clothing or flick them off skin. If they are attached, it's imperative that the ticks be removed without leaving their heads embedded in the skin. Do not traumatize the tick or squeeze its body in the center. Either use a tick scooper — a plastic device available from your vet for little more than a dollar — or sterile tweezers to grab the tick as close to the head as possible. Pull the tick straight out and use the tweezers to remove any part left in the wound. Afterward, wash the area and your hands well with antiseptic soap and water, dry, then apply a few drops of infection-fighting echinacea tincture.

Follow-Up Care for Bug Bites

If you have lots of itchy bites, any one of the following ingredients added to a warm bath may provide some relief:

- 1 cup (230 ml) apple cider vinegar
- 1 pound (454 g) baking soda (use half as much for children)
- 1 gallon (3.8 l) infused tea of peppermint, white oak bark, or cleavers
- ½ cup (115 ml) sea salt
- 1 cup (230 ml) cornstarch

TICKS AND DISEASE

Ticks have been a cause for special concern in the past few years due to their ability to transmit Lyme disease. The longer an infected tick remains attached, the greater the chance for infection. Symptoms of Lyme disease, which can take from two days to two weeks to manifest, include arthritis-like symptoms such as achy joints, chills, rashes, facial palsy, headaches, swollen glands, fatigue, numbness, irregular heart rhythms, and a bitemark that resembles a bull's-eye. The longer Lyme disease remains undiagnosed, the more difficult it is to treat.

In addition, a tick pathogen, *Rickettsia rickettii*, is known to cause Rocky Mountain spotted fever. Symptoms of Rocky Mountain spotted fever, which may appear one week after a tick bite, include intense headache, itching, a rash on the ankles and wrists, and fever.

As a precaution, if you are bitten by a tick, take 1 dropperful of echinacea or red root tincture 3 times daily for a few days to give the immune system a boost. You might also want to drink calendula and cleavers teas. Calendula is antiseptic and helps treat infections deep in the body, while cleavers reduces fever.

If despite your precautions, you suspect you have contracted Lyme disease or spotted fever, visit a health-care professional.

Prevention of Bug Bites

Mosquitoes and other insects are repelled by many natural substances. They include:

- **Homeopathic Staphysagria.** Taking 4 pellets dissolved under the tongue 4 times daily a few days prior to an outing may discourage mosquitoes from biting you.

- **Essential oils.** A drop or two of cedarwood, citronella, lavender, and tea tree essential oils can be applied topically to pulse points such as the inside of the wrists, behind the knees, and behind the ears every hour or so to repel buzzing bombers. If you don't have essential oils, you may rub aromatic plants such as artemesia, lavender, or rosemary on your body. See the box below should you wish to make your own insect repellent blend.

- **Garlic.** Taking a 500-mg garlic capsule 3 or 4 times a day will make you an unappetizing target for anything that bites.

- **Diet.** Avoid large amounts of sugars, alcohol, and tropical fruits and juices when you know you're going to be outdoors. Some people feel that these items attract bugs.

- **Aromatherapy.** Place a few drops of citronella, eucalyptus, geranium, lavender, rosemary, or tea tree essential oil in a diffuser to discourage flying insects. You can also mix a glass of water with about 30 drops of the oil to use as a room spray.

- **Tomato leaves.** Hang a bouquet of dried tomato plant leaves in the room to repel mosquitoes.

HERBAL INSECT REPELLENT

Instead of soaking your body with a potentially dangerous chemical, try this natural insect repellent that encourages insects to choose another target. You can make up a bottle before mosquito season, and keep it handy in the refrigerator all summer long.

- ¼ cup (58 ml) almond or sunflower oil
- 5 drops *each* of eucalyptus essential oil, lavender essential oil, tea tree essential oil, citronella essential oil, and rosemary essential oil

BURNS

First-degree burns leave a painful red mark without blisters and often occur from brief contact with a hot object. Mild sunburn is a first-degree burn. Only the first layer of skin is affected.

Second-degree burns develop blisters and swelling. They are more painful, deeper, and may appear wet. There may be raw, red blisters. They may be caused by boiling water or contact with a very hot object, such as a woodstove. A severe sunburn could be classified as a second-degree burn. They are more likely to cause scarring than are first-degree burns.

Third-degree burns may look white and charred. They may be caused by electrical shock or prolonged contact with a hot object. Since skin and nerve endings are often destroyed, the pain may actually be less than with a first- or second-degree burn, but there is a greater likelihood of infection. Third-degree burns are frequently surrounded by lesser-degree burns that will probably be painful.

Seek immediate medical attention if:

- A large area of skin is burned (more than 10 percent in a child or 15 percent in an adult)
- The burned area develops blisters or swelling
- The burn has resulted from severe electrical shock
- The burned area is on the face
- The eyes are burned

While you wait for medical attention:

- **If the eyes have been burned by fire,** flush with cold water.
- **If the eyes have been burned by chemicals,** flush with cool water for a full five minutes, then refer to *Eyes — Heat and Chemical Burns* on page 53.
- **If the face is burned,** keep the injured person sitting or propped up and observe carefully for breathing difficulty.

- **If a large area is burned,** do not apply cold water or ice as this can cause further shock. Instead, help the burned individual lie down on a sheet or rug, then cover the burned area with a clean sheet or other material that is not fluffy.

- **In the case of white, charred burns (third-degree burns),** do not apply water or even remove clothing. Wrap the area in a cold, wet cloth, and take 4 pellets of homeopathic *Cantharis,* dissolved under the tongue.

- **Provide electrolytes** (available at most health food stores; see also recipe on page 47).

- **Treat for shock** (see page77).

At-Home First Aid for Burns

At-home first aid is appropriate only for first-degree burns. Remove rings or tight clothing near the burn since they may be difficult to remove if swelling occurs.

Cool the burn to prevent further damage to the skin. Fill a basin of cold, not freezing, water and submerge the burned area in it for as long as it takes for the pain to subside. Should water be scarce, rinse with milk or beer or apply clean, wet compresses. Never apply anything to a burn before cooling it in water (or milk or beer) as you can actually seal in the heat, which will cause more damage.

After cooling the burn, there are several simple treatments to soothe and help heal the burned area:

Household and herbal remedies.
Essential oils. After cooling the burn, either lavender or tea tree essential oil can be applied undiluted to the burned area to relieve pain, promote healing, and prevent infection.

Aloe. Keep a jar of aloe vera gel on hand in the refrigerator; aloe is the perfect remedy for relieving pain, preventing infection, and promoting healing. Or you can simply pull off and split the lower leaves of an aloe plant and apply the sticky inner gel.

Poultices. Poultices made of comfrey, grated carrot, tofu, raw potato, and plantain can help cool inflammation and promote healing.

Tea bags. Cooled black tea bags can be used the same way as poultices — plus they have the advantage of being quicker and easier to make.

St.-John's-wort. An oil, lotion, or salve made with St.-John's-wort can be applied regularly to the burned area to encourage healing.

Quick kitchen remedies. Spread raw honey or yogurt over the burn to cool inflammation and promote healing.

Homeopathic remedies. For immediate shock, administer 2 drops of Rescue Remedy, under the tongue or mixed in 1 cup (230 ml) of water. Then give 4 pellets, dissolved under the tongue, of the appropriate remedy for the situation.

Urtica urens can be given when an agonizing pain that feels like stinging occurs.

Hypericum can be used internally to help repair nerves damaged by burns.

Arsenicum album can be used for burned skin that is scaly, red, swollen, and sensitive to touch.

Chinese medicine. A Chinese patent formula for burns is Jing Wan Hong (also known as Ching Wan Hung), which can be topically applied after the burn has cooled. Just smear onto clean gauze and bandage or tape in place over the burn. Change and reapply the bandage daily as necessary. *Note:* This remedy can discolor clothing, so wrap it well.

Follow-Up Care for First-Degree Burns

Burns that increase in pain more than two days after the incident, discharge pus, or cause problems with joint movement should be seen by a health-care professional. If a fever develops, the burn should also be checked whether or not any other symptoms occur.

Fluids. Drink plenty of fluids, especially water and fresh juices, to prevent dehydration. Cucumber juice is especially cooling.

Elevation. To help alleviate pain and swelling, keep the burned area elevated.

Cold pack. An insulated, dry, cold pack can help relieve pain.

Herbs. To help the body heal, make a tea (see page 128) using 2 parts comfrey leaf, 1 part red clover blossoms, 1 part nettles, 1 part skullcap, and 1 part marshmallow root. Drink ½ cup (115 ml) every 2 hours for up to 3 weeks.

Swallow one 500-mg capsule each of comfrey root (to promote cell regeneration) and echinacea (to prevent blood poisoning or infection) every 2 hours for 3–4 days.

Nutritional support. Eat high-protein foods such as spirulina, chlorella, and blue-green algae as they contain protein to rebuild damaged tissues. Traditional Chinese medicine encourages eating crab and mung bean soup to help heal by reducing heat in the body.

Supplements. Burn victims are prone to candida, so use an acidophilus supplement to minimize fungal growth. Take antioxidants such as beta carotene, vitamin C, vitamin E, and zinc to promote healing and minimize scarring.

Protection. Shield any burned areas from the sun. Avoid applying anything with cotton balls, which have irritating fibers that can stick to the burn.

Follow-Up Care for Second- and Third-Degree Burns

In addition to the guidelines for follow-up care of first-degree burns, there are some additional techniques useful for treating more serious second- and third-degree burns. Avoid breaking blisters or removing tissue. Soak burned areas in salt water to promote healing.

A classic formula for the treatment of second- and third-degree burns is to blend ½ cup (115 ml) wheat germ oil with ½ cup (115 ml) raw honey and ½ teaspoon (2.5 ml) lobelia powder. Store the mixture in a clean glass jar in a cool place. When needed, add enough chopped or blended comfrey leaves to make a paste. Gently apply with a sterilized paintbrush. (To sterilize the brush, immerse it in boiling water for 1 minute.) Don't clean the paste off the burn, but paint on additional layers 2 or 3 times daily to regenerate new skin.

CHEMICAL CONTAMINATION
(See also *Eyes — Heat and Chemical Burns*)

Seek immediate medical attention for all chemical contamination.

While you wait for medical attention:

- **If the chemical was a dry agent,** protect your hands with rubber gloves, then brush as much of the chemical as possible away from the victim. Use a soft brush or duster. Remove contaminated clothing and rinse the person with cool water. Be sure to position the person so that the poison is not washed onto another part of the body.

- **If the chemical was wet,** remove any contaminated clothing and then rinse the victim repeatedly with plenty of cool water for about 10 minutes.

- **If the chemical was inhaled,** get the victim into fresh air as soon as possible. Open windows, get her outside, do whatever it takes. Encourage the individual to breathe deeply and evenly. Loosen tight clothing. If possible, stop the source of the fumes by turning off the car, stove, or any other possible source.

Follow-Up Care

After an episode of poisoning, eat foods high in pectin such as apples and carrots, which will help flush out remaining contaminants. Drink 1 teaspoon (5 ml) of green clay dissolved in 1 cup (230 ml) of water daily for 2 weeks; the clay will absorb toxins and then will be excreted. Eat a low-fat diet to help prevent poisons from being absorbed deeper into the body. And include miso soup and seaweed in your diet — both contain substances that will bind with some chemical residues and carry them out of the body.

Protect Yourself!

If you must enter a contaminated area while trying to rescue someone, here's how to protect yourself:

- Protect your lungs by covering your nose and mouth with a wet cloth

- Take several deep breaths before entering the contaminated area

- Stay low, avoiding vapors if possible

Milk thistle seed can help protect the liver from absorbing poisons. Take two 500-mg capsules 3 times daily for several weeks following the poisoning episode.

Shiitake and Reishi mushrooms are helpful *adaptogens*, substances that help the body acclimate to stress. Take two 500-mg capsules of either one (or 1 capsule of each) 3 times daily for several weeks.

You may also want to drink teas made with purifying herbs such as burdock root, dandelion root, and red clover blossoms. Drink 3–4 cups daily for several weeks following the poisoning episode.

CHOKING

Seek immediate medical attention if:

- Any foreign object obstructing the airway cannot be dislodged
- The individual is not breathing
- The individual's breathing is noisy
- A bluish color appears around the lips and ears
- You are forced to perform the Heimlich maneuver

While you wait for medical attention:

Encourage the person who is choking to cough — this may be enough to dislodge any blockage. If she is having trouble coughing or breathing, ask if she is choking:

- **If she can cough or speak,** let the individual attempt to expel the blockage without help.
- **If she can't cough but is breathing,** the airway is partially obstructed. Arrange for immediate transport to an emergency medical facility to remove the blockage.
- **If she cannot speak, cough, or breathe,** the individual is choking. Get someone to call for medical help while you perform the lifesaving Heimlich maneuver (see page 11).

Follow-Up Care for Choking

After the blockage has been expelled or removed, a cup of slippery elm or marshmallow root tea or papaya juice will soothe an irritated throat.

CUTS (See *Abrasions and Lacerations*)

DIAPER RASH

At-Home First Aid

Diaper rash can be caused and aggravated by diapers left on too long, plastic pants, food sensitivities, and yeast growth. Here's what you can do to relieve your baby's discomfort and heal his or her bottom:

Household remedies.

Exposure. Expose the baby's bottom to fresh air by laying him or her on the diaper rather than fastening it. When the baby does wear diapers, change them frequently. Avoid disposable diapers, and avoid rubber or plastic pants.

Apple cider vinegar. If you launder your own cloth diapers, add ¼ cup (58 ml) apple cider vinegar to the final rinse water.

Diet. Diaper rash may occur when either the mother's or baby's diet has become overly acidic. It may indicate that tomatoes, citrus products, sweets, and even fruits are being overconsumed or are otherwise aggravating. Try reducing amounts of these foods first. If that doesn't work, talk to your doctor about eliminating them completely.

Ointment. The pharmacy favorite, vitamin A & D ointment, is a safe and effective treatment. Follow the package instructions.

Calendula. Salves or teas made with calendula can be applied to soothe the irritation and promote healing. Apply after every diaper change.

Yogurt. Plain, raw yogurt can also be applied to soothe and help heal the rash.

Prevention of Diaper Rash

Consider giving your baby an acidophilus supplement that is specifically formulated for infants. If you're nursing, you may also want to use an acidophilus supplement designed for adults. Acidophilus is a friendly bacteria that naturally occurs in yogurt; it will help replenish friendly intestinal flora.

DIARRHEA

Seek immediate medical attention if the individual:

- Has blood in his or her stool
- Vomits
- Has dry, sticky saliva
- Has dark, concentrated, or scanty urine
- Has a temperature of 103°F (39°C) or more with a fast pulse, lethargy, and sunken eyes
- Does not improve within a week (or within 24 hours, if an infant)

While you wait for medical attention:

Give frequent sips of water or, if available, an electrolyte beverage (see page 47). Avoid drinking juices.

At-Home First Aid

Diarrhea is often nature's way of eliminating something that probably shouldn't be in the body in the first place. That's why it's always best to try and determine the cause of the problem. Possible causes include: viruses, bacteria, intestinal parasites, side effects from medication, overuse of laxatives, and food intolerance. It is common for people to experience cramping along with the runs. Here are a few suggestions for soothing the intestinal tract while it's under attack:

Fluid therapy. Diarrhea can often lead to dehydration, so increase fluid intake. Make sure the beverage is at room temperature, and drink in small sips. Following are some healing formulations.

- 1 teaspoon (5 ml) of *carob powder* blended into 1 cup (230 ml) of spring water is an excellent remedy that can be used for children as well as adults

- 1 teaspoon (5 ml) *green clay* mixed with 1 cup (230 ml) water

- The following *teas* are recommended: blackberry leaf (for mild cases of diarrhea), blackberry root (for stronger cases), strawberry leaf (especially good for infants), or cinnamon bark, raspberry leaf, or white oak bark.

- A spoonful of *slippery elm* powder and a pinch of *ginger* powder mixed with a cup of hot water, taken every hour or two, will help relieve symptoms.

> ## Electrolyte Rehydration Drink
>
> Whenever someone's been dehydrated by illness or injury, make them an electrolyte-rich beverage by adding ⅛ teaspoon (1.3 ml) each of baking soda and sea salt to 8 ounces (230 ml) of water.

Household remedies.

Diet. Try the BRAT diet. BRAT is an acronym for Bananas, Rice, Applesauce, and Tea or burnt Toast. Other beneficial foods include yogurt with active cultures, cooked carrots, miso soup, and oatmeal.

Charcoal absorbs toxins. Take two 500-mg charcoal capsules every 2 hours (while you're awake) to stop even the most stubborn cases. Continue treatment for a day or two after diarrhea has stopped.

Umeboshi plum paste. Stir 1 teaspoon into a cup of hot water and drink every 2 hours (while awake — discontinue while sleeping). Take an additional 3 times daily for 1–2 days after diarrhea has stopped.

Supplements.

Psyllium seed. Although it's usually used as a laxative, psyllium can solidify the stool. Take two 500-mg capsules 3 times a day or stir 1 rounded teaspoon (5 ml) of psyllium into a bit of water.

Electrolytes. Since diarrhea causes a loss of minerals, use an electrolyte supplement from a natural food store. Follow dosage instructions on the package.

Acidophilus. An acidophilus supplement may also help by encouraging your intestine to recolonize itself with friendly bacteria that will help prevent future problems. Again, follow dosage instructions on the package.

Homeopathic remedies. Take 4 pellets dissolved under the tongue 4 times daily of the appropriate remedy for the situation described.

Arsenicum album. Use for food poisoning and sudden onset conditions in which the affected individual is restless, so weak he or she wants to lie down, and doesn't want to be left alone. Other indications: The individual is worse in early morning or after midnight, and feels chilled and thirsty but only drinks small amounts of water at a time. Sometimes the stool is acidic and irritates the rectum. The individual may also vomit, especially after consuming food or drink.

Nux vomica. Use when the affected individual is irritable and oversensitive to light, noise, and odor; when food poisoning is suspected; or when the diarrhea has been brought on by overindulgence in food or alcohol. Other indications: The individual may complain of chills, have poor appetite, and feel worse in the morning. There is usually abdominal cramping. Elimination gives temporary relief, but the stool is scanty and contains mucus.

Phosphorus is indicated when diarrhea is copious and without pain. Other indications: The patient is weak, very thirsty, inclined to vomit, and easily startled. He or she may also have night sweats.

Podophyllin is often used for sudden onset children's diarrhea when it is painless yet profuse. The stools are often watery and yellowish-greenish with a bad odor. The condition is often aggravated by teething, eating, a fruit binge, moving around, or overexcitement.

Sulphur is indicated for diarrhea that is worse at 5 or 6 A.M. The odor is sulfurous, like rotten eggs, and the anal area may be irritated.

For children, I suggest *Chamomilla* (2 pellets dissolved under the tongue 4 times daily). It's especially useful in cases of children who are irritable and want to be held. Other indications: The diarrhea was brought on by fear and nervousness; the child is usually worse in the evening; one cheek may be red, the other pale; the diarrhea is often greenish with mucus.

Chinese medicine.

Acupressure. Massaging around the navel for two minutes in a circular motion is an effective acupressure technique.

DROWNING

> Seek immediate medical attention for all rescued drowning victims.

While you wait for medical attention:

1. **If the individual is not breathing, begin CPR.**

2. **Once the individual is breathing,** turn the victim onto his or her side in the recovery position.

3. **Rub the feet, hands, and ears to encourage good circulation.** Keep the individual warm. Do not administer food or drink.

4. **If the patient is conscious consider homeopathic remedies,** if they're available. Rescue Remedy is helpful for shock — 2 drops under the tongue. Try four pellets dissolved under the tongue of any of the following for the particular conditions described:

   Antimonium tartaricum for near drowning when the victim is bluish and cold, covered with sweat and has rattling breath

   Aconitum for shock, fear

   Arsenicum for fear and anxiety

5. **When the patient revives, offer ginger tea.** Once the patient is conscious and breathing easily, ginger tea can help warm the body and calm nausea.

Follow-Up Care

Following the instructions on the bottle, take garlic and ginkgo supplements for a few days following an almost-drowning episode. Garlic will help prevent a lung infection and ginkgo helps the body better utilize oxygen.

DRUG/ALCOHOL OVERDOSE (See also *Alcohol Poisoning*)

Seek immediate medical attention if the individual:

- Has a slow pulse
- Has difficulty breathing
- Has paled in complexion and is sweating
- Cannot be roused
- Is vomiting
- Is diabetic
- Has taken drugs with alcohol

While you wait for medical attention:

1. If breathing stops, check the airway for an obstruction and begin CPR (see page 3).

2. If the individual convulses, do not administer anything or induce vomiting. After convulsions have subsided, place the individual in the recovery position (see page 18) so fluids can drain from his or her mouth.

3. Ask the victim what they have taken as soon as possible in case they lose consciousness.

- **If the victim is conscious,** give 1 teaspoon (5 ml) of charcoal in a glass of water.
- **If the victim has overdosed on alcohol, barbiturates, tranquilizers, or opiate derivatives** and is conscious, also give him or her strong black tea or coffee as a stimulant.

4. Loosen clothing to help keep the airway open. Open a window to allow fresh air in.

5. Keep the individual calm. Keep him or her away from crowds, bright lights, intense movement, and loud sounds, all of which can worsen the crisis.

6. Gather a sample of any vomit, drugs, syringes, or containers associated with the overdose. Give it to medical personnel when they arrive.

Follow-Up Care for Drug/Alcohol Overdose

To prevent a hangover: Take one teaspoon of honey or a 100-mg B-complex tablet before bed and upon arising. Drink plenty of fluids. A shot of angostura bitters in the morning will also help.

EAR INJURY

Seek immediate medical attention if:
- Any part of the ear is detached
- The victim cannot hear from one or both ears
- Fluid is leaking from the ear

While you wait for medical attention:

1. Elevate the victim's head.

2. If the eardrum has been perforated, place a clean piece of gauze in the *outer* ear to provide protection. Do not clean the ear or stop any fluid from leaking out.

3. If there are any wounds, lightly apply a dressing using even pressure.

4. Place the individual on his or her injured side to allow fluid to drain. Place a small pillow under the head and shoulders.

Follow-Up Care

If an infection develops, check with your doctor and consider taking echinacea every couple of hours while you're awake — 1 dropperful of tincture, 1 cup (230 ml) of tea, or two 500-mg capsules.

ELECTRIC SHOCK

Seek immediate medical attention!

Remember, electric burns may be deeper than what is apparent on the skin. Even a tiny burn mark can indicate serious injuries.

While you wait for medical attention:

Check to see if the victim is breathing. If he or she is not, tilt the victim's head to open the airway and begin CPR (see page 3).

Follow-Up Care

Treat the person with 1 dropperful of black walnut tincture, given orally 3–4 times daily for 3–4 days. Black walnut contains ellagic acid, which may help people recover from electric shock by stimulating the nervous system.

Four pellets of homeopathic *Phosphorus* can be taken, dissolved under the tongue, every half hour for 2–3 days after the shock to help the patient, who may be weak, fearful, and anxious.

BREAKING THE CIRCUIT

The most important point to remember is this: Don't touch someone who is still in contact with an electric current! You could get shocked as well. Here are some tips for approaching the victim of an electric shock so you can begin first aid.

- Turn off the electricity by pulling the plug or shutting down the circuit that affects the outlet involved.
- Be careful not to step in any liquids, including the victim's urine, which can conduct current.
- Be aware that simply pulling the plug may not shut off the electricity. Before you pull the victim away from whatever caused the shock, make sure you are standing on something insulated and dry such as a thick book, rubber mat, blanket, newspaper, or wooden box.
- Do not touch the victim until the current is broken. If you're not sure whether or not the circuit is broken, use a long, nonconducting item like a stick, branch, dry rope, towel, or anything else that isn't metal, doesn't contain metal, and isn't damp to help remove the victim from the source of electricity.

EYES — HEAT AND CHEMICAL BURNS

Seek immediate medical attention if:

The victim complains of a burning sensation in his or her eyes

While you wait for medical attention:

1. Flush the affected eye with a gentle stream of water for at least 5 minutes. Do not rub. Do not pause to remove contact lenses. If the victim does wear contacts, simply engage the drain stopper so that the contacts don't wash down the drain. If just one eye is contaminated, make sure the victim's head is tilted with the contaminated eye down. That way, chemicals will not be washed from one eye to the other.

2. If the victim's eyes have been burned by an acid, flush the eyes a second time with a solution of 1 teaspoon (5 ml) baking soda in 1 quart (920 ml) of water.

3. After rinsing, cover the affected eyes with a clean, dry cloth or bandage. Do not use cotton balls, which can leave particles in the skin.

4. If the victim's eyes have been burned by heat, such as from spitting fat or fire embers, follow the instructions above, then cover both eyes with a cold water compress.

Follow-Up Care

The homeopathic remedy *Euphrasia* may also help heal any inflammation — take 4 pellets 4 times daily for 2–3 days.

FAINTING

Seek immediate medical attention if the individual:

• Does not regain consciousness within 5 minutes

• Is known to have a serious health condition

• Is elderly

While you wait for medical attention:

1. Place the person who fainted in the recovery position (see page 18).

2. Periodically check the individual's breathing and heart rate. Should either stop, begin CPR (see page 3).

At-Home First Aid for Fainting

When someone faints but does not need immediate medical care, here's what to do:

Elevation. Raise the individual's feet 8 to 12 inches (20 to 30 cm). Turn his or her head to one side and position it lower than the heart.

Comfort. Loosen tight clothes. Apply cold, moist towels to the neck and face. Do not slap or shake the victim — and don't throw water at him.

Fresh air. When well-meaning people crowd around, ask them to move back so the person who fainted can get fresh air.

Aromatherapy. To bring someone out of a faint, sprinkle a few drops of either lavender, peppermint, or rosemary essential oil on a clean cloth, hold it under the victim's nose, and tell them to sniff. Or wave a freshly cut onion under his nose.

Homeopathic remedy. A few drops of Rescue Remedy, the Bach flower remedy for shock and trauma, can be placed behind the victim's ears or on the lips or wrists. If they are conscious, a few drops of Rescue Remedy can be taken in water or directly under the tongue.

Prevention

If someone complains of feeling faint, have the person lie down (preferably) or bend over with his or her head to or between the knees. Pinch the fleshy skin between the upper lip and nose using a slightly upward pressure (it's an acupressure point that awakens the heart).

If the individual is fainting from heat, try rubbing an ice cube on his or her wrists. Have the person lie down in a cool place and drink cool liquids.

FEVER

Seek immediate medical attention if:

- A child has a fever over 103°F (39°C) that lasts for over twelve hours
- A child or adult has a fever of 105°F (41°C)
- A pregnant woman has a fever over 102°F (39°C)

While you wait for medical attention:

Place the individual in a cool (96°F [36°C]) bath.

At-Home First Aid

Fever is actually an ally. It heats the body until it fries invading bacteria. So don't try to lower a fever unless it's higher than 103°F (39°C), because the body is simply doing its job to destroy viruses and bacteria.

Caution: Do not give aspirin to someone who has the flu or chicken pox. It can increase susceptibility to Reye's Syndrome (a condition affecting mostly children that causes abnormal liver and brain function). When you do need to lower fever, here are some nonaspirin natural alternatives:

Household remedies.

Fluids. Keep the person hydrated with plenty of cool water. If you like, add a few slices of fresh lemon — its crisp clean scent always makes people feel better, and it has a cooling effect. If the person has been sweating or had diarrhea, give an electrolyte-rich beverage (see page 47) or oatstraw tea.

Soaks. Soak the individual's feet in cool water.

Herbal remedies.

Compresses. Prepare cool compresses and add five drops of peppermint or lavender essential oil. Apply them to the groin area, wrists, and neck, and then use them to sponge the individual's hot body.

Teas. Offer teas of elder flower, ginger, peppermint, and yarrow, all of which are diaphoretic (they help to increase perspiration), which will help the body cool down.

FOOD POISONING

Seek immediate medical attention if:

- Nausea, vomiting, or diarrhea persists for longer than three days
- There is blood in the stool
- Dehydration becomes severe (symptoms include lack of urination, sticky saliva, rapid pulse, and sunken eyes)

While you wait for medical attention:

1. Keep the individual warm.

2. Offer fluids.

At-Home First Aid

If food poisoning is not an emergency, any one of the remedies below will help alleviate the symptoms of nausea and diarrhea:

Household remedies.
Vinegar and honey. Mix 1 tablespoon (15 ml) each of apple cider vinegar and honey into 1 cup (230 ml) of warm water and drink. Repeat every 2–3 hours.

Charcoal. Take two 500-mg charcoal capsules mixed with 1 cup (230 ml) of water. Repeat every 2–3 hours. (This treatment may make the stool look black.)

Green clay. Mix 1 teaspoon (5 ml) of green clay in a cup of water and drink. Repeat every 2–3 hours.

Umeboshi plum paste. Mix 1 teaspoon (5 ml) in a cup of water and drink. Repeat every 2–3 hours.

Herbal remedies. Ginger or peppermint tea will help calm the stomach.

Follow-Up Care for Food Poisoning

When the individual feels like eating again, offer him or her small amounts of easily digested foods such as miso soup, broth, applesauce, or yogurt.

Acidophilus can help recolonize the digestive tract with healthy bacteria; take 1 capsule 3 times daily, 30 minutes before meals, for 2 weeks. Garlic can help kill any lingering pathogens acquired from eating the tainted food. Taking a dropperful of echinacea tincture 2 times daily and boosting vitamin C intake for a few days after recovery can help protect against food poisoning in the future.

FRACTURES

Seek immediate medical attention if:

- An area of injury appears swollen, misshapen, and/or discolored
- The injured individual is unable to move or has great pain upon moving or touching the area
- You or the injured person heard or felt a bone snap

While you wait for medical attention:

1. Immobilize the injured area. Use a splint or sling, if possible (see page 16). Move the victim as little as possible. Don't attempt to reset a bone yourself. If a bone is protruding, don't attempt to push it back into place. Once the limb is splinted, it may be elevated to help control the bleeding.

2. Do not allow the individual to eat or drink. He or she may need surgery. Recently ingested food and liquid can be life threatening while the individual is under anesthesia. Ask when he or she last ate so that you can relay the information to medical personnel should the victim lose consciousness.

Follow-Up Care for Fractures

Follow-up care is designed to help rebuild bone. Besides eating well-balanced, high-protein meals, you might consider calcium, magnesium, and essential fatty acid supplements. Teas of nettles, oatstraw, horsetail, and raspberry leaf may also help. And you might consider the homeopathic *Ledum* for the first 2–3 days, followed by 2–3 days of homeopathic *Symphytum* (for each, 4 pellets dissolved under the tongue 4 times daily). To aid in healing, apply comfrey daily, in the form of a poultice or salve, to the injured area; cover with a hot, moist towel and leave on for 30 minutes.

FROSTBITE (See also *Hypothermia*)

Areas furthest from the heart — the feet, hands, nose, ears, and face — are most at risk for developing frostbite. The early stage, called *frostnip,* manifests as numbness and tingling. As the skin freezes further it may become white, grayish, glossy and pale, or bluish. Blisters can appear. Pain may be felt early on, but later subside. Consider extreme frostbite a medical emergency.

Seek immediate medical attention if:
- The skin becomes white, grayish, glossy and pale, or bluish
- Blisters appear
- The person with frostbite cannot walk
- Frostbitten areas cannot be protected from further cold exposure
- A frostbitten area does not improve with one half hour of indoor treatment

While you wait for medical attention:

1. Cover any frozen part.

2. Get the victim indoors. Remove jewelry, watches, and any constrictive clothing. (*Caution:* If the frostbitten area is in danger of freezing again before medical attention is available, do not attempt to thaw it out.)

3. Let your skin warm theirs. If the individual's fingers or toes are frostbitten, place these appendages in a warm place such as in your armpit or between your thighs. Do not use radiant or dry heat, such as from a lamp, because it can warm the affected area too quickly. Do not rub or massage frostbitten areas, as doing so may cause tissue damage.

4. If frostbite is in the mild (incipient) stage, the affected member can be rewarmed by placing the frozen part in water that is 105–110°F (41–43°C). Use the milder temperature for children. Offer the homeopathic remedy *Apis* for burning and stinging pain as the area is being warmed. If warm water is inaccessible, gently wrap the affected area in a warm blanket or sheet.

5. After warmth has returned to the area, cover the area with a cloth, then with a blanket or sleeping bag.

6. Offer something warm to drink (avoid alcohol or caffeinated beverages). Ginger tea is ideal.

7. Once circulation has been reestablished, the area may become itchy, red, and painful. Stop warming at this point. Swelling is likely to develop after thawing and further warming will only make the swelling worse.

8. After the frostbitten body part has been rewarmed, flex or exercise it if possible.

9. Do not break any blisters that form.

Follow-Up Care for Frostbite

After medical assistance has been rendered, here's how to help the affected area heal:

Household remedies.
  Chile pepper. Crush 1 teaspoon (5 ml) of chile peppers into ½ cup (115 ml) of sesame oil and apply to the skin to improve circulation to the area. Avoid mucous membranes.

Niacin. Ask your doctor about taking 100 mg of niacin. It will dilate capillaries and veins, thus improving circulation to the affected skin.

Supplements. Vitamin C (1,000 mg), vitamin E (400 IU), coenzyme Q10 (50 mg), zinc (25–50 mg), and bromelain (500 mg), each taken 2 times daily, can reduce inflammation, speed healing, increase circulation, and prevent infection. Note: Bromelain must be taken 1 hour before meals or at least 3 hours after, or it acts as a digestive enzyme and loses its anti-inflammatory properties.

Herbal remedies.

Essential oils. Mix 5 drops geranium, ginger, or eucalyptus essential oil in 1 teaspoon (5 ml) vegetable oil and gently apply to the skin.

Ginger. The day after the frostbite crisis, take a ginger tea bath. To prepare, simmer, covered, 8 teaspoons (40 ml) dried or 1 pound (454 g) fresh ginger in 2 gallons (7.6 l) of water for 20 minutes. Strain out the liquid and add to a full tub.

Aloe. Apply aloe vera gel to frostbitten areas to help tissue repair.

Homeopathic remedies. Take 4 pellets, dissolved under the tongue, 4 times daily of the appropriate remedy:

Arnica for the shock and trauma

Agaricus for frostbite with cold, tingling numbness, or feeling like the affected area is being pierced by ice needles

Lachesis for feet that appear blue or purplish

Hypericum for nerve damage

HEAD INJURY (See also *Bleeding*)

Seek immediate medical attention if the injured person:
- Has cold, clammy skin or a flushed face
- Has a rapid, weak, or slow pulse
- Is dizzy, dazed or faint or loses consciousness
- Has difficulty breathing, or her breathing seems noisy

- Has extreme thirst
- Is bleeding from the ears or nose, or is coughing up blood
- Has a severe headache
- Has a fluid discharge from either ear
- Has pupils of different sizes
- Convulses
- Is weak, uncoordinated, has difficulty speaking, or suffers some sort of paralysis

While you wait for medical attention:

Do not give food or liquid, other than to moisten the lips with water. If the individual is conscious, give 2 to 4 drops of Rescue Remedy under the tongue. If he or she is not conscious, apply Rescue Remedy to the wrists or behind the ears.

Follow-Up Care for Head Injury

Observe the victim for at least the next 24 hours for signs of disorientation, irritability, unequally dilated pupils, and lack of muscle control in the mouth. If any of these symptoms appear, seek medical attention.

Homeopathic *Natrum sulphuricum* (4 pellets dissolved under the tongue 4 times daily) is good for head injuries where mental capabilities have been impaired. Also consider taking 1–3 teaspoons (5–15 ml) daily of the supplement lecithin, which is rich in nutrients for the brain and nerves.

To repair memory and mental functions after a head injury, both calamus and rosemary essential oil are good aromatherapy remedies. Place a few drops in an aromatherapy diffuser, add 5–7 drops to a bath, or 15 drops to ½ cup (115 ml) of carrier oil for a massage.

HEART ATTACK

A heart attack occurs when the supply of oxygen-rich blood to the heart is cut off. *It can be fatal.*

Seek immediate medical attention if the individual shows any symptoms of a heart attack. These include:

- Lightheadedness or loss of consciousness
- Uncomfortable or crushing chest pain or pressure
- Shortness of breath
- Heavy sweating
- Pain beneath the sternum, sometimes spreading to the shoulders, arms, neck, and jaw
- Confusion
- Pale or bluish tint to skin
- Anxiety and fear of death

While you wait for medical attention:

1. If the victim has been prescribed medication for just such an occurrence, help them take it.

2. Have the victim lie down. Prop up his or her head and shoulders with pillows, but don't move unnecessarily as it will strain the heart. Make the person comfortable by loosening his or her clothing, especially around the neck, chest, and waist.

3. Encourage the individual to breathe deeply and slowly.

4. Keep the individual warm. Provide good ventilation but avoid chilling drafts.

5. Don't allow him to eat or drink.

6. Bite firmly but gently down on the outsides of both of the victim's little fingers. This stimulates the heart meridian and can help open up blockages.

7. If the individual is fully conscious, offer 1 dropperful of cayenne tincture mixed in 1 cup (230 ml) of water every 5 minutes until help arrives. Cayenne helps block pain and stimulate blood circulation.

8. If the individual becomes unconscious, place them in the recovery position (see page 18).

9. If the person stops breathing or if their heart stops, give CPR (see page 3).

HEAT STROKE

Seek immediate medical attention if the individual:

- Is disoriented
- Has a headache
- Has a strong, rapid pulse
- Is dizzy
- Has a high body temperature
- Has hot, dry skin
- Loses consciousness

> ### Caution
> *Heat stroke can be fatal.* If you suspect an attack of heat stroke, seek immediate medical attention!

While you wait for medical attention:

1. Place the victim in the recovery position (see page 18).

2. Start cooling the person down. Bathe the individual's bare skin with cool water and fan vigorously with anything available.

3. Make cool compresses. Soak washcloths in cool water (if you have them on hand, add 5 drops of lavender or peppermint essential oil to the sink). Put one on the back of the victim's neck and one under each armpit.

At-Home First Aid for Overheating

First aid for overheating is the best way of preventing heat stroke. If you suspect that the heat is getting to you, try some of the following simple preventive treatments.

Cool down. Get into the shade, lie down with your head elevated, and loosen your clothes.

Make a spritzer. Fill an 8-ounce spray (230 ml) bottle with water, 2 teaspoons (10 ml) of witch hazel, 10 drops of lavender essential oil, and 10 drops of peppermint essential oil. Spray or sprinkle over yourself.

Rehydrate. Drink a pint of water to which a pinch of salt has been added, or ask someone to make you a rehydration drink (see page 47 for recipe). After that, drink something every ten minutes. Do *not* drink caffeinated beverages. Hibiscus flower, lemon balm, oatstraw, and peppermint tea are all cooling beverages, especially when chilled. Or simply squeeze lemon or lime into water for a cooling effect.

Homeopathic remedies for overheating are:

Veratrum album for weakness, clammy skin, nausea, and dizziness

Carbo vegetabilis for the exhausted person who seems ready to collapse

Byronia for a splitting headache due to overexposure to heat accompanied by excessive thirst and dry throat

Gelsenium for heat that leaves the individual dizzy, weak, and drowsy

Glonoine for hot, sweaty skin with a throbbing headache

Magnesia phosphorica for heat exhaustion where spasms occur in the abdomen, arms, and legs

Prevention of Overheating

- Nosh on cucumbers and watermelon, both of which contain lots of water, to keep you from getting dehydrated.
- Keep potassium levels up with a hot weather diet rich in avocados, bananas, cantaloupe, and potatoes.

• If hot weather is new to you, Siberian ginseng in capsules, tincture, or tea may help you acclimate.

• Boost your vitamin C intake.

• Avoid alcoholic beverages.

HIVES

Hives are an allergic response. They are frequently the first indication that someone is having a life-threatening reaction to a medication or an herb.

Seek immediate medical attention if the individual:

• Has difficulty breathing

• Becomes weak

• Experiences nausea

• Develops facial swelling

While you wait for medical attention:

1. Think. Ask the victim if he or she has any known allergies. Do your best to figure out what caused the allergic reaction. Prevent further ingestion or contact.

2. If breathing is impaired, reach for ephedra. If the individual is having problems breathing and is exhibiting the symptoms listed above, he or she is having a severe allergic reaction. Give 2 dropperfuls of ephedra tincture to dilate bronchioles and prevent anaphylactic shock. In emergencies of severe allergies, take in addition a dose of 1 teaspoon (5 ml) baking soda mixed in a glass of water to alleviate symptoms. *Caution:* Ephedra should not be used by those taking medication for heart conditions or high blood pressure. Ephedra should be used with caution by those suffering from angina, diabetes, glaucoma, heart disease, high blood pressure, enlarged prostate gland, or overactive thyroid gland — do not exceed the recommended dosage!

At-Home First Aid for Hives

As long as you do not need to seek immediate medical attention, the following may help reduce itchiness and swelling:

Household remedies.
Oatmeal. Tie a couple of handfuls of oatmeal into a washcloth, toss it into your bath, then soak in the tub until the water cools. Pat onto your skin any oatmeal mucilage that oozes out.

Cornstarch. Dust your body or the affected area with cornstarch to keep the skin dry and cool.

Herbal remedies.
Tea. Drink calendula, chamomile, dandelion leaf and root, nettles, plantain, or red clover tea.

Aloe. Apply aloe vera juice to the hives after bathing and drying off.

HYPOTHERMIA (See also *Frostbite*)

Hypothermia, which is brought on by exposure to cold, wind, or rain, lowers the body's temperature to the point that vital organs can no longer function. The brain is one of the first organs affected.

Seek immediate medical attention if the individual:

- Develops stiff muscles or loses consciousness
- Slurs his speech
- Stumbles or acts as though he is irrational, confused, or intoxicated
- Has sudden bursts of energy followed by fatigue
- Develops a headache
- Develops blurry vision
- Develops abdominal pains

While you wait for medical attention:

1. Get the individual out of the weather.

2. Remove any wet clothing and replace with dry.

3. **Insulate individual** with whatever's available — sleeping bag, extra clothing. Make sure the head is covered.

4. **Apply hot water bottles to groin and sides of torso** (high heat-loss areas).

5. **Handle individual carefully** and move no more than necessary.

6. **If individual is conscious, offer sips of hot, sweet liquids.**
Note: Do not rub or massage an individual with hypothermia.

Follow-Up Care for Hypothermia

Offer sweet hot drinks such as spiced cider or ginger tea, but not alcohol or drinks containing caffeine, both of which affect the cardiovascular system. Then, as the individual is able to eat, offer cooked, warm foods such as soup and oatmeal. Since garlic and ginger improve circulation, use them liberally in whatever you prepare. Avoid cold foods such as salad.

INSECT BITES (See *Bug Bites* and *Stings [Bee, Hornet, and Wasp]*)

JELLYFISH STINGS

Anaphylactic shock is possible from jellyfish stings.

Seek immediate medical attention if you experience any of the symptoms of an allergic reaction:
- Nausea
- Difficulty in breathing
- Difficulty swallowing
- Fever
- Heart palpitations

While you wait for medical attention:

1. Prevent further stinging by brushing away tentacle fragments.

2. Scrape off any remaining stinging cells with a sharp-edged object such as a credit card. A towel will suffice if nothing else is available.

3. Rinse with sea water, not ever with fresh water.

4. Neutralize the sting. Apply up to 5 drops of lavender essential oil to help neutralize the sting. Reapply every 15 minutes. (Urinating on the stung area will have the same effect.)

5. Start healing. Apply vitamin E or aloe vera juice to heal tissue and reduce inflammation.

Follow-Up Care for Jellyfish Stings

Taking 1 dropperful of echinacea tincture 3 times daily for 1–2 days and boosting your vitamin C intake can reduce inflammation and help the body neutralize any toxins.

NETTLE RASH

At-Home First Aid

It is widely believed that wherever nettles grow, a remedy to soothe their sting is close at hand. Here's what some of them are and how to use them. Chop any of the following herbs, mix with a bit of water, and apply as a poultice. In an emergency, simply chew the herb and apply it to your skin.

- Jewelweed leaf
- Mint leaf
- Mullein leaf
- Plantain leaf
- Rosemary leaf
- Sage leaf
- Yellow dock leaf

NOSEBLEEDS

Seek immediate medical attention if:

- Blood flows from both nostrils and doesn't stop for 20 minutes
- The nosebleed has occurred after a head injury
- The bleeding lasts for longer than half an hour despite applications of cold and pressure
- The bleeding resulted from a severe blow that also caused dizziness and nausea
- The nose looks crooked or displaced in any way
- The individual is elderly
- The individual has high blood pressure
- The individual is using blood-thinning drugs

While you wait for medical attention:

1. Sit down and lean forward. Have the individual lower her head and leave her mouth open. Try to stop the bleeding by pinching the soft part of the nostril closed by pressing with the thumb and index finger, below the cartilage, for at least ten minutes. Release the pressure slowly.

2. Loosen any clothing around the neck.

3. Apply a cold water compress to the base of the skull and top of the nose to help constrict blood vessels. After ten minutes gradually release the nostrils, but still sit quietly and avoid blowing the nose for at least three hours.

> ### Tip
>
> To calm a frightened child who has a nosebleed, sprinkle 2 drops of lavender essential oil on a tissue and have the child hold the tissue to his or her nose.

At-Home First Aid

If the nosebleed does not require medical assistance, try to stop the bleeding with the "While you wait" steps above. If they prove unsuccessful, try any of the following remedies.

Household and herbal remedies.

Apple cider vinegar. Snuff a bit of apple cider vinegar diluted in water — the strength of the solution will depend on your tolerance for it.

Cayenne. Drinking ⅛ teaspoon (.6 ml) cayenne powder mixed in a cup of warm water can help stop the bleeding.

Cold water. Drinking plain cold water can help stop a nosebleed.

Yarrow leaf. Place a pinch of crushed yarrow leaf in the nostrils.

Homeopathic remedy. Four pellets, dissolved under the tongue, of the homeopathic remedy *Ferrum phos* may help curb profuse bleeding.

Follow-Up Care for Nosebleeds

Most nosebleeds don't last longer than 15 minutes. Take it easy and rest for at least half an hour afterward. Avoid vigorous exercise for a day or two so that the nose doesn't start bleeding again. Avoid tobacco smoke since it can dry out the nasal passages and make them prone to bleed.

Prevention

If you frequently get nosebleeds, check with your doctor. Consider taking a supplement of vitamin C with bioflavonoids, and add doses of nettles or shepherd's purse (1 dropperful of tincture 3 times daily) to strengthen the capillaries and promote healthy blood clotting.

If your nose bleeds due to excessive dryness, apply a bit of herbal salve inside your nose. Consider placing humidifiers in your home and work environments.

POISONING (See also *Food Poisoning*)

Seek immediate medical attention for all poisoning! Symptoms may include:

- Dizziness
- Nausea
- Headache
- Impaired speech
- Visual disturbances
- Chest pains
- Convulsions
- Paralysis

While you wait for medical attention:

1. Call your local poison control center. Have the poison container in your hand when you call. Be prepared to give the approximate weight and age of the person poisoned. Try to find out if they have vomited. If there is a sample of vomited material, scoop it into a container and hold it — along with the poison container — for medical personnel.

2. Do not induce vomiting, unless directed by poison control and never in an unconscious person. Vomiting up strong acids, strong alkalis, and petroleum products can burn the esophagus and airway and be inhaled and absorbed into the lungs. Burns around the lips are a sign that these products have been ingested.

3. If the poison control center suggests you help the victim vomit, give syrup of ipecac with lots of water. The standard dose is 1 tablespoon (15 ml) for children and 2 (30 ml) for adults followed by 1 or 2 cups (230 or 460 ml) of water. Repeat in 20 minutes if vomiting doesn't occur. Sticking a finger or spoon in the back of the throat can also induce vomiting. Vomiting is often recommended for noncorrosive substances such as toxic plants and most drugs.

4. After vomiting, give the person 1–2 tablespoons (15–30 ml) activated charcoal in a glass of water to adsorb remaining poisons. Since charcoal can adsorb even the syrup of ipecac, do not administer charcoal until after vomiting has occurred.

5. If the poison control center suggests diluting the poison rather than vomiting, give the victim lots of water or milk. Have them drink slowly so as not to induce vomiting.

6. If the poison control center suggests using an absorbent material, give 1–2 tablespoons of activated charcoal mixed in 1 cup (230 ml) of water.

Prevention of Poisoning

Most poisoning fatalities occur in children between the ages of one and three. Aside from keeping chemicals and medicines out of their reach, here's how we can help keep them safe:

- Avoid taking medicine in front of kids. They love to imitate parents.

- Mark containers with poisonous materials clearly. That may not stop the child, but at least we'll be able to tell medical personnel what he or she ingested.

- Never put food or drink in bottles or jars that once held toxic substances.

- Don't store chemicals and medicines on the same shelves as food.

- Store all medicines and chemicals in a locked cabinet.

Quick Fix

A universal antidote for poisoning is:

2 parts burnt toast (charcoal to adsorb toxins)

1 part milk of magnesia (alkaline to offset acids)

1 part strong black tea (tannic acid to offset alkaline)

Check with your poison control center before using this formula.

POISON IVY, OAK, AND SUMAC (See also *Hives*)

Reactions to poison ivy, oak, and sumac may occur any time between 6 and 72 hours after exposure. Be alert for signs of an allergic reaction, as they can be life threatening.

Seek immediate medical attention if:

- The victim's throat swells
- The victim experiences cramps, diarrhea, nausea, or vomiting
- Hives appear near the eyes, mouth, or genitals
- Hives cover more than half the body
- The victim develops a high fever

At-Home First Aid for Poison Ivy, Oak, and Sumac

If you think you've contracted poison ivy, oak, or sumac and you do not need immediate medical attention, here's how to minimize its affects:

1. Clean the affected area(s). Remove your clothing and toss it in the washing machine as soon as you realize you've been exposed. Then take a shower. Use an alkaline soap without an oil base, such as Fels Naptha soap, to avoid spreading the urushiol. Avoid washing with a washcloth, as this will cause the oil to spread.

2. Apply topical relief.
   Teas. A tea made from burdock leaf and root, calendula, goldenseal root, grindelia, myrrh, plantain leaf, or white oak bark can be used topically to reduce itching and swelling. Chop up a bit of any of the above herbs, steep, covered, in simmering water for 5–15 minutes (as long as you can wait!), then strain and apply to the affected area. For long-term use, put 1 cup (230 ml) of the herb in a large glass or stainless steel container. Cover with boiling water. Cover and let stand 12 hours. Strain the tea and apply the liquid to the afflicted area.

   Jewelweed juice. Another excellent herb for topical use is jewelweed (*Impatiens* spp.), which is rich in natural tannins that help reduce inflammation. Simply run the fresh herb through a juicer or blender, collect the juice, and dab it on the affected areas every 2–3 hours. Since jewelweed is only available during the summer months, and poison ivy, oak, and sumac are available far longer, freeze the jewelweed juice into ice cubes and store it in plastic bags in the freezer. Apply the juice or frozen cubes directly to the skin.

   Poultice. A poultice can also be made of green clay or grindelia and apple cider vinegar.

> ## What Got You
>
> The toxic principle in poison ivy, oak, and sumac is called urushiol. It is one of the most potent toxins on earth. Its toxicity can persist for years after the plant is dead. One-quarter ounce (7 g) of urushiol has the potential to affect everyone on earth!

Follow-Up Care for Poison Ivy, Oak, and Sumac

If you do develop hives after coming into contact with one of these plants, don't scratch! You may find that bathing brings some relief when you add 1 cup (230 ml) of apple cider vinegar, oatmeal, baking soda, or cornstarch to the bathwater.

Liquid Swedish bitters, available at health food stores, is also helpful. It is designed to be a digestive aid, but, used topically, it dries the hives quickly.

There are also a number of topical home remedies that can help relieve and speed healing of "the awful itch." Here are just a few:

- Mix water with cornstarch, baking soda, oatmeal, or Epsom salts to form a paste. Apply to blisters and let dry.
- Apply aloe vera juice, tofu, or watermelon rind.
- Whisk 1 tablespoon (15 ml) sea salt into a pint of buttermilk and apply to the skin.
- Use homeopathic *Sulphur* (dissolve 4 pellets under the tongue 4 times daily) for burning itch worsened by warmth, with severe itching that makes you scratch until you bleed.
- Apply fresh urine to the affected skin. It's true — human urine can work wonders on an itchy case of poison rash.
- Help cleanse your system by drinking herbal teas. Some good choices would be burdock, dandelion root, nettle, and red clover.

Prevention

The wisest precaution is to learn to identify the plant and avoid it. Wear gloves and clothing that covers you well before going out in infested areas. One folk remedy for prevention is to rub fresh artemesia leaves on exposed skin when going out. Many people find that homeopathy can help them better resist poison ivy. Try:

Rhus tox (which by the way, is made from poison ivy). Three pills can be dissolved under the tongue, every 2 hours before exposure.

Anacardium 3x. Five pellets dissolved under the tongue each day can be taken for 5 days before exposure.

Ledum. Four pellets dissolved under the tongue 4 times daily can be used right after exposure to prevent a rash from occurring.

SCORPION STINGS

Seek immediate medical attention if:

- The victim experiences nausea, fever, dizziness, muscle spasms, or breathing difficulty
- The bite is from the sculptured scorpion (commonly found in the southwestern United States)

At-Home First Aid

If immediate medical attention is not needed, wash the wound with soap and water. Watch for any breathing difficulty and swelling — both signs of anaphylactic shock. Remedies to help heal the bite:

Lavender. Dab a few drops on the bite every hour as needed for 2 or 3 days.

Echinacea. Dab a few drops of the tincture on the bite every hour as needed for 2 or 3 days. It's also beneficial to drink a tea made from the dried or fresh herb.

Garlic. Apply mashed garlic to a scorpion bite for 10 minutes. (Any longer can irritate the skin.)

Lime. Cut a fresh lime in half, squeeze some juice on the bite, then apply the cut face of the lime to the bite for 10 minutes.

Rest. Take it easy for at least twelve hours.

SEIZURES OR CONVULSIONS

Seek immediate medical attention if:

- Seizures last longer than five minutes, or happen consecutively
- The victim does not regain consciousness between seizures
- The victim is pregnant
- The victim is having difficulty breathing
- The seizure happens when the individual is in the water

While you wait for medical attention:

1. Help the victim lie on the floor and clear a space around him. Do not restrain him since holding a seizing person down can result in injury. Despite what you may have heard, don't put anything in the victim's mouth.

2. Place a soft pillow under the head as a cushion. Loosen clothing and remove glasses.

3. Monitor breathing. If the individual stops breathing, begin CPR (see page 3).

4. Monitor the seizures. Time the duration of the seizure, and if there is more than one, keep count of how many. Relay this information to medical personnel when they arrive.

At-Home First Aid for Seizures or Convulsions

When the individual comes out of the seizure, give him comfort and reassurance. Stay with him until he's fully recovered. Suggest that he rest as you do the following:

Massage. Rub the earlobes firmly for a few minutes to stimulate acupressure points.

Acupressure. Apply upward pressure to the fleshy skin between the upper lip and nose (it's an acupressure point that awakens the heart).

Rescue Remedy. Do not give anything to drink until the individual is alert, then give him a couple of drops of Rescue Remedy either alone or in a few ounces of water.

Prevention

Chlorella, an edible micro-algae, is a good food supplement for people prone to seizures as it provides oxygen for the brain. Try one or two 500-mg capsules 3 times daily. Other super supplements to use on an ongoing basis are calcium, magnesium, taurine (an amino acid), B complex, and lecithin. Black cohosh, catnip, and skullcap are antispasmodic herbs.

Eat healthfully and avoid aspartame, other sweeteners, and foods contaminated with heavy metals. Avoid camphor and sage essential oils, as in rare cases they may trigger a seizure.

Practice yoga breathing techniques for relaxation and keep your vertebrae in proper alignment by practicing good posture.

SHOCK

Shock results from suppression of the body's vital systems through injury or illness. Heart and respiration rates go up, while blood vessels become constricted. Rough handling of an injured person or delayed treatment for an injury can exacerbate the symptoms of shock. Even if an injury or illness does not seem severe, shock can be fatal.

Seek immediate medical attention if an injured or ill person develops:

- Cold, clammy, pale, moist skin
- A rapid (over 100 beats per minute), faint pulse
- Irregular breathing
- Thirst
- Weakness and nausea
- Restlessness and anxiety
- Disorientation and incoherent talking

> **Caution**
>
> Do not move anyone with a possible head, neck, or spine injury.

While you wait for medical attention:

1. Check breathing and heart rate. Be prepared to administer CPR if it becomes necessary (see page 3).If breathing becomes labored or the individual vomits, place the individual into the recovery position (see page 18).

2. Help the victim lie down. Loosen clothing at chest, neck, and waist. If the individual becomes unconscious or has severe wounds of the jaw or lower portion of the face, turn the victim on his or her side to drain oral fluids and prevent choking.

3. Elevate the feet 8–12 inches (20–30 cm) using a folded coat or whatever else is handy. This will facilitate breathing and blood circulation.

4. Slightly elevate the head (unless you suspect a head or neck injury). Lower it if the victim complains of chest pain.

5. Keep the person warm. Cover only enough to prevent the body from losing heat.

6. Hold the individual's hand and reassure them. Avoid panic and loud noises.

If the person is conscious, there are several soothing liquid formulations you might offer them. Adults can ideally be given about ½ cup (115 ml) every 15 minutes until medical assistance arrives. Children (ages 1 to 12) should take ¼ cup (58 ml) and babies under a year ⅛ cup (29 ml) over a 15 minute period. If victim gets nauseous or vomits, discontinue fluids. Some of the choices include:

Rehydration drink. A solution of ½ teaspoon (2.5 ml) of baking soda and 1 teaspoon (5 ml) salt to 1 quart (920 ml) of water.

Any hot, sweet liquids. However, do not offer fluids to those with head or abdominal injuries. Do not leave the victim to get fluids — send someone else.

Rescue Remedy (2 drops under the tongue), rock rose (Bach flower essence, 2–4 drops under the tongue), or homeopathic *Arnica* (4 pellets dissolved under the tongue). These are calming emergency remedies to administer.

Aromatherapy. Waft aromatic, centering essential oils or crushed herbs such as lavender, rosemary, or peppermint under the person's nose.

SNAKEBITE

A bite from a poisonous snake can be fatal!

Seek immediate medical attention if you have been bitten by a poisonous snake.

Signs of poisonous snakebite include:

• Bruising or swelling

• Sharp pain around a bite of one or two puncture wounds

• Nausea, vomiting, or diarrhea

• Blurry vision

• Breathing problems, convulsions, or seizures

While you wait for medical attention:

1. Wash the area with soap and water. Wipe outward, away from the wound.

2. Remove the venom. If you have a snakebite kit, use the suction cup to remove the venom, preferably in the first five minutes after the bite occurred, before the venom starts circulating. Do not use your mouth to suck out venom as you could end up being poisoned. Do not cut into the flesh. Remove constrictive items such as rings, bracelets, or shoes as swelling may occur.

3. Apply ice. If ice is not available, place the limb in a cool stream. Immobilize the bitten area and keep it at or below the heart level.

4. Use any strip of cloth to make a constricting bandage — *not* a tourniquet. Apply a constricting band for pit viper bites 2 inches above the bite. Make sure it is not tight and that a finger can easily be slipped underneath the band. Loosen the band every fifteen minutes.

5. Give the victim fluids to drink (but not alcohol).

6. Keep the victim calm. Agitation increases blood flow, bringing the venom into the bloodstream. If the victim must walk any distance, make sure it is very slowly.

7. Monitor the victim's airway. Be ready to administer CPR if necessary.

Follow-up Care for Snakebite

Follow-up treatments for snakebite focus on neutralizing the venom and boosting the body's antibodies. Here are some suggestions:

Echinacea. Use echinacea orally and topically. Give 1 dropperful of echinacea tincture every hour for up to 12 hours following the bite. Saturate a gauze pad with echinacea tincture and apply to the bite. Echinacea tincture stimulates the production of the white blood cells that neutralize the venom.

Vitamin C. Give 1,000 mg vitamin C every 2 hours to help stimulate the body's production of natural antibodies.

Homeopathic Arnica. This remedy can be good for the trauma of it all.

Poultices. A salt pack moistened with vinegar or a green clay and apple cider vinegar poultice can be applied as drawing agents.

Garlic. Eat it fresh to remedy snakebite or take it in capsules as an antiseptic agent.

> ## Common Sense Beats Copperhead
>
> Years ago I was bitten by a copperhead snake, many miles away from a hospital or even telephone. Fortunately, we did have electricity. My husband, without missing a beat, turned on the vacuum cleaner and sucked the venom out with the wand. Just goes to show that sometimes you need to improvise!

SPIDER BITES

Seek immediate medical attention if the victim:

- Has difficulty breathing
- Goes into shock
- Experiences nausea, vomiting, or convulsions
- Has a history of allergic reactions to insect bites
- Has increasing pain
- Is a young child

While you wait for medical attention:

1. Immediately wash the bitten area.

2. Keep the bitten area lower than the heart to slow down assimilation of the spider's venom. Icing the bitten area will also help.

3. Neutralize the venom. Depending on what you have on hand, topical application of any of the following quick remedies will help neutralize the venom and help the tissues heal:

- Three to five drops lavender essential oil
- Apple cider vinegar
- Mashed garlic clove (apply for no more than 10 minutes to avoid skin irritation)
- A few drops of St.-John's-wort tincture and vitamin E oil

At-Home First Aid for Spider Bites

The steps and remedies listed above for use in an emergency situation will also provide relief for nonvenomous but itchy or painful spider bites.

SPRAINS AND STRAINS

Sprains occur when a ligament or tendon (tissues connected to the muscles and bones near a joint) is stretched beyond its normal range of motion. Strains occur when muscles are stretched beyond their normal range. Both result in pain and swelling.

Seek immediate medical attention if:

- Pain or swelling from an injury is severe
- A fracture is suspected
- A joint is swollen or out of alignment
- Loss of sensation occurs in any part of the body

While you wait for medical attention:

The trick to remembering how to treat sprains and strains is this: R.I.C.E. The letters stand for Rest, Immobilize, Cold, and Elevation.

1. Rest. Sit down, get ready to immobilize, ice, and elevate, and be sure to rest the injured limb for a couple of days.

2. Immobilize. Move the injured area as little as possible.

3. Cold. Apply a cold compress to help constrict the blood vessels, which will minimize bleeding and swelling. A good compress can be made by mixing 1 tablespoon (15 ml) arnica tincture or homeopathic *Arnica* oil with 1 pint (460 ml) of cold water, then soaking a cloth with the solution and applying it to unbroken skin over the injured area. If the area begins to feel numb from the cold, remove the compress until the numbness subsides. Then reapply. Repeat for at least 6–12 hours following the injury.

4. Elevation. Keep the injured area higher than the heart to minimize swelling.

At-Home First Aid for Sprains and Strains

If you're sure the injury is not a medical emergency, follow the instructions above. Then try these remedies to reduce swelling and speed healing:

Household and dietary remedies.
Cold compresses. In addition to cold water or ice, cold compresses can be made with apple cider vinegar, tofu, chopped comfrey, plantain, green clay, cabbage, chopped onion, grated raw potato, tea tree essential oil, burdock, or ginger tea. A solution of apple cider vinegar mixed with sea salt can be gently applied to the area.

Herbal liniment. A liniment for sprains can be made by stirring 1 tablespoon (15 ml) cayenne pepper and ½ teaspoon (2.5 ml) birch essential oil into a pint of apple cider vinegar. Apply topically to inflamed area 3–4 times daily.

Phytochemicals. Eat foods rich in the phytochemical anthocyanadin — blackberries, blueberries, cherries, and raspberries, for example. They'll strengthen blood vessels and muscles.

Supplements. Take a 500-mg calcium and 1,000-mg magnesium supplement to keep muscles supple. Boost your intake of vitamin E (to help oxygen utilization) and potassium (to bring energy to the cells). A 500-mg dose of bromelain 3 times daily can help reduce pain and swelling. Two 500-mg capsules of turmeric 3 times daily for 2–3 days may help reduce inflammation.

Homeopathic remedies.

Byronia is used when the injury is hot, red, and swollen. Pain is worse with movement and the injury needs to be held tightly.

Ledum is for sprains that are purple and puffy. The injury feels cold, yet cold compresses bring relief.

Rhus tox is for sprains that feel worse when initially moved, but better after repeated motion.

Ruta graveolens is for old sprains that are worse from being still and better with movement.

Prevention of Sprains and Strains

When the injured area has been pain free for at least ten days, light exercise can be reinstated. To help prevent these injuries in the future, stretch for at least ten minutes before athletic activities.

STINGRAY STINGS

At-Home First Aid

A stingray has venomous spines in its tail. One flick next to your leg while you're wading along the Florida coast, and you'll find out just how painful they can be. Here's what to do if a stingray leaves one of its spines in your leg:

1. Carefully remove the barb if it is still embedded.

2. Soak the affected area for 20 minutes in a saltwater or hot-water bath to help break down the neurotoxin the barbs release.

3. Neutralize the sting. After soaking, make a paste of baking soda and water or baking soda and apple cider vinegar and apply to the stung area. Papaya powder — the main ingredient in meat tenderizer — can also be mixed into a paste and applied to break down the venom.

Follow-Up Care for Stingray Stings

To help prevent infection and stimulate healing, use tincture of echinacea internally, 1 dropperful 3 times daily for 1–2 days.

Prevention

To avoid running into a stingray, give it fair warning that you're around. Stingrays bury themselves under the sand in shallow areas of coastal waters, so make sure you shuffle your feet when walking in the shallows.

STINGS (Bee, Hornet, and Wasp)

Stings can be fatal. If you experience any of the signs of an allergic reaction listed below, seek immediate medical attention!

Seek immediate medical attention if:
- The individual's tongue swells
- The individual is wheezing or has difficulty breathing
- You observe skin flushing or a sudden-onset rash
- The individual develops a severe cough
- The individual complains of blurred vision
- The individual vomits or complains of nausea

While you wait for medical attention:

1. Remove the stinger. Being careful not to squeeze the venom sac at the base of the stinger, gently pull out the stinger by dragging the edge of the fingernail across the imbedded stinger in the direction opposite from its entry. If this is ineffective, use tweezers. Remove the stinger as quickly as possible as the venom sac can release poisons for two or three minutes.

2. If the individual is allergic, inject epinephrine, if available. If (and only if) the individual is allergic, check to see if she is carrying a special "pen" that injects epinephrine. Many people who know they are allergic to beestings carry them. The epinephrine will help dilate the airway and prevent anaphylactic shock.

At-Home First Aid for Stings

Remove the stinger, clean the wound, then stop pain and swelling:

1. Extraction. Remove the stinger as directed in step 1 above.

2. Cleansing. Wash the area with soap and water.

3. Find relief. Try any of the remedies listed below.

Garden remedies. Some of the simplest topical remedies that relieve pain and swelling can be found right at your feet. They include: mud, green clay, and freshly chewed plantain leaf.

Kitchen remedies. Other remedies to reduce pain and swelling are found in your kitchen. Try:

Meat tenderizer (papain powder). Mix with water into a paste and paint over the wound with your fingers.

Baking soda. Mix with vinegar into a thick paste and plop it on the wound.

Onion. Cut fresh slices and lay over the wound.

Cold milk. Dip a clean cloth in milk, wring out, fold, and apply.

Herbs. A dropperful of echinacea tincture taken 3 times daily can help reduce swelling. Two drops of lavender essential oil or moistened tobacco leaf are also effective when applied topically to neutralize the venom.

Homeopathic remedies. All homeopathic remedies should be taken internally by dissolving 4 pellets under the tongue.

Apis is ideal for stings that cause redness, hot and rapid swellings, and pain that is worsened by heat.

Vespa is for stings from wasps.

Follow-Up Care for Stings

One thousand to 5,000 milligrams of vitamin C and 100 milligrams of pantothenic acid up to 5 times during the day for the first day help provide a natural antihistamine effect, thus reducing swelling. Other supplements to consider:

- **Bromelain,** an enzyme derived from pineapple, will help relieve swelling. Take one 500-mg capsule 3 times daily for 1–2 days.
- **Quercetin** is a flavonoid with anti-inflammatory properties. Take one 500-mg dose every 4 hours for 1–2 days.

Prevention

If you're allergic to beestings, carry an emergency epinephrine "pen" at all times. Discuss with your health care provider if you think you need one.

If you're attacked by an angry swarm of bees, hornets, or wasps, run into thick bushes or jump into a body of water — if, that is, you can swim!

STOMACH PAIN (See also *Food Poisoning*)

Seek immediate medical attention if you are experiencing symptoms of appendicitis:

- Spasms in abdomen — pain is usually felt at the navel but also in the lower right side of the abdomen
- The stomach is tender to the touch, movement worsens pain, and sleep may be difficult
- Vomiting
- Breath may smell foul
- Temperature is around 102°F (39°C)

Caution

Never apply heat to stomachaches of unknown origin. Heat can cause the appendix to rupture in cases of appendicitis.

While you wait for medical attention:

1. Do not allow the victim to eat.

2. To alleviate pain and inhibit toxicity, try one or more of the following, if the ingredients are available:

- Give 1 dropperful of echinacea tincture every 2 hours.
- Dip half of a toothpick in ume concentrate; dissolve the concentrate in a cup of chamomile tea and drink.
- Apply a cool castor oil compress over the inflamed area.

3. Rinse the mouth with sips of water, but if you suspect appendicitis avoid drinking.

4. Keep the patient quiet in a semi-sitting position.

At-Home First Aid for Stomach Pain

If you're sure the individual does not need medical assistance, in addition to the remedies outlined above, a few simple teas can often ease the pain. Try agrimony, slippery elm, chamomile, peppermint, or ginger.

STROKE

Seek immediate medical attention if you experience any symptoms of stroke, including:

- Sudden headache
- Paralysis or numbness on either or both sides
- Difficulty swallowing, breathing, or speaking
- Difficulty seeing
- Dizziness or loss of balance
- Loss of bladder or bowel control
- Confusion
- Loss of consciousness.

While you wait for medical attention:

1. If the person is unconscious, place them in the recovery position (see page 18).

2. If the person is conscious, help him or her to lie down. The head should be slightly higher than the feet.

3. Loosen clothing around the neck, chest, and waist.

4. Keep the victim cool to minimize damage. Try fanning them and applying cold water compresses to the wrists, neck, and pelvic area.

5. Do not give food or drink.

6. Monitor breathing. Be prepared to administer CPR if necessary (see page 3).

Follow-Up Care for Stroke

Treatment can include cerebral tonics such as the herbs ginkgo or gotu kola (one to two 500-mg capsules or 1 dropperful of tincture 3 times a day), the antioxidant lipoic acid (one 1,000-mg capsule), and the essential fatty acid DHA (according to label specifications), as part of a daily nutritional protocol.

SUNBURN (See also *Burns* or *Heat Stroke*)

At-Home First Aid

Here's how to soothe the burn:

Household remedies.

Rehydration. Drink plenty of water to rehydrate the skin.

Soaks. Soak in a tepid bath. Add 1 cup (230 ml) of apple cider vinegar, 1 cup (230 ml) of black or green tea, or 7 drops of peppermint or lavender essential oil. Or add ½ cup (115 ml) of baking soda and a small handful of sea salt.

Yogurt. Blend yogurt and cucumber and apply to the skin. Leave on for 20–30 minutes, then rinse off.

Milk compress. Soak a clean cloth in cold milk. Squeeze out excess liquid and apply to burned area.

Herbal remedies.

Aloe juice. Add a few drops of lavender essential oil to aloe vera juice and smooth over your skin.

Peppermint. Drink peppermint tea to cool you from the inside.

Chamomile poultices. For sunburned eyes, apply damp, cooled, chamomile tea bags as a poultice.

St.-John's-wort. Apply an oil or cream made with St.-John's-wort. *Caution:* Do not expose skin to further sun, as St.-John's-wort can increase sun sensitivity.

Homeopathic remedies. Depending on the situation, try 4 pellets dissolved under the tongue 4 times daily of the appropriate remedy:

Cantharis for burns with blisters relieved by cold compresses (do not break blisters); also helps minor sunburn

Urtica urens for minor sunburn

TOOTHACHE

At-Home First Aid

Every toothache needs to be checked by a dentist. Until you can see one, however, try the following remedies to quell the pain.

Household remedies.

Salt water. Add 1 teaspoon (5 ml) of salt to 1 cup (230 ml) of water (hot or cold) and swish it around in your mouth. Repeat every couple of hours.

Garlic. Place a piece of garlic on the tooth for about an hour.

Ice. Put small pieces of ice in your mouth.

Herbal remedies.

Essential oils. Apply 2 drops of clove or tea tree essential oil on the tooth and surrounding gum area. For children and for those who prefer a milder solution, dilute the clove oil with equal parts vegetable oil or vodka.

Poultice. Apply a plantain poultice.

Pine resin. Apply resin from a pine tree.

Ginger compress. Apply it to the cheek area over the afflicted tooth.

Herbal foot bath. A hot ginger or mustard tea foot bath will help to draw pain away from the head. Soak your feet for 3 minutes in hot tea, then plunge them into icy cold water for 1 minute. Alternate back and forth for about 15 minutes, always beginning with the hot and ending with the cold.

Valerian. Take two 500-mg valerian capsules up to 3 times daily.

Homeopathic remedies. Dissolve 4 pellets of the appropriate remedy under the tongue 4 times daily.

Belladonna can help reduce the swelling and pain of a rapid onset infection in the early stages.

Hepar sulph helps to drain pus from an infected abscess.

Chamomilla is for severe toothaches in which the person is sensitive to heat and feels worse at night. People who need this may have a low pain threshold. Pain sometimes radiates toward the ear.

Coffea is for intense stinging pain that is worse from chewing and warm drinks.

Magnesia phosphorica is for intense piercing pain shooting along the tooth's nerve. The pain improves when cold water is in the mouth.

Staphysagria should be used when major decay is causing the pain.

Chinese medicine.

Acupressure. Apply pressure using a rapid, circular massage to the tips of your index fingers on each side of the nail.

UNCONSCIOUSNESS (See also *Fainting* and *Head Injury*)

Seek immediate medical attention for all cases of unconsciousness.

While you wait for medical attention:

1. Check for breathing. If the individual is not breathing, begin CPR (see page 3).

2. If the victim is breathing, check to see if they are responsive. Ask: "Are you okay?" Gently tap or shake. Do not harshly shake or slap the person as this could aggravate spinal or neck injuries.

3. Treat for bleeding if necessary (see page 31).

4. If you are absolutely certain there is no spinal injury, place in the recovery position (see page 18).

5. Rub the individual's ears to stimulate acupressure points. Call to them.

6. Do not give an unconscious person anything to eat or drink as it could cause choking.

7. Crush some aromatic herbs and wave them in front of the individual's nose. Lavender or peppermint essential oil are also effective.

8. In a firm voice, command the individual to breathe and awaken.

9. Prevent shock by keeping the individual warm.

VOMITING
....

Seek immediate medical attention if vomiting:
• Causes uncontrollable dehydration

• Lasts for more than 24 hours

• Is excessively violent

• Smells like feces

• Is dark green or brown

While you wait for medical attention:
Follow any of the suggestions outlined under At-Home First Aid.

At-Home First Aid

If you do not need medical attention, try any one of these remedies:
Household remedies.

Lemon. Suck on a piece of lemon.

Ume. Try some ume concentration in a bit of water, or 1 teaspoon (5 ml) umeboshi plum paste in 1 cup (230 ml) of water.

Ginger ale. Sip some real ginger ale made from the herb.

Compress. An apple cider vinegar compress can be applied to the abdomen to curb vomiting.

Herbal remedies. Drink peppermint or ginger tea.
Homeopathic remedy. Four pellets of *Nux vomica* dissolved under the tongue can help relieve emergency digestive ailments.
Massage. Rub the stomach gently in a counterclockwise direction.
Acupressure. Press on the acupressure point for nausea. It is located in the middle of the inner forearm, two-and-one-half finger widths above the crease of the wrist.

Acupressure point for nausea

WOUNDS
....
(See *Abdominal Injuries, Abrasions and Lacerations, Bleeding*)

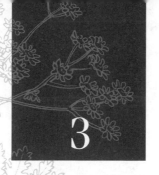

SURVIVING NATURE'S CHALLENGES:
Tips and Techniques for Emergencies

Accidents considered minor mishaps at home can easily evolve into dangerous situations when they occur away from phones, cars, and clean running water. Such is often the case after natural disasters or when you're traveling in the wilderness. Preparation is your most important ally. In the event of a natural disaster, loss of power, or encounter with a wild animal, you will want to initiate concrete action, not fumble through a book looking for answers or search aimlessly for supplies. If you've read through the information and prepared yourself, both with supplies and knowledge, you'll be well equipped to handle the situation.

AVALANCHE

Signs of an avalanche can include cracking ice sounds, snowballs that roll downhill, and white clouds and dust uphill. If you see any of these signs, head sideways rather than downhill. If you are on skis and at the avalanche edge, try to ski out. If it's too late to ski out, get rid of encumbrances such as backpacks or skis. As the avalanche overcomes you, take in a big breath, close your mouth, and cover your nose to prevent snow from entering the lungs and throat and causing suffocation.

Hang on to the downhill side of any fixed object such as a rock pinnacle, as the avalanche may keep flowing past you. If you get swept downhill, *swim* against the tide toward the nearest edge. Use either the backstroke, breaststroke, or dog paddle. If necessary, use your arms to fend off slabs of snow and rocks, but keep trying to get to the surface by swimming.

Once the slide has stopped, use every effort to break out of the snow immediately as it will set up hard within minutes. Wrap both arms over and around your head to create breathing space. When you've stopped moving, quickly make as large a cavity around you as possible to allow for air space before snow freezes, which happens quickly. Then try to dig yourself out. Should you end up buried, determine which way is up by collecting some saliva in your mouth and dribbling it off your lips. If the spit moves toward your nose, you'll know that you are upside down. If breathing is difficult, conserve oxygen by minimizing movement and breathing slowly. Survival is possible under the snow for some time.

If you're carrying a whistle use it to signal, or shout when you hear people.

To prevent getting caught in an avalanche to begin with, never go onto mountain slopes within 24 hours of a big snow, or during warm-weather intervals and spring thaws.

Sun and heat can cause avalanches, so travel only on slopes that have already had sun exposure and are holding solidly. Slopes with lots of trees and irregular surfaces are often at a lower risk for avalanche. If you need to traverse a dangerous slope, travel in a party and cross one at a time, roped together, so that others know where you are and can help should a rescue prove necessary.

On long trips, have a professional guide who knows the area accompany you. And if you venture into the snowy winter wilderness, make sure you carry a shovel strapped to your backpack as well as an electronic locating device.

BEAR

Should you meet a bear, don't run away. The bear can run faster. Instead, stay calm and do not make any sudden moves.

If you run into a bear with cubs, slowly back away at an angle, keeping your eye on the bear while talking in an even tone. If the bear isn't moving and there's a tree you can climb, move slowly toward it. Drop anything you're carrying — it will make climbing easier and may distract the bear. Grizzlies won't climb higher than ten feet (three meters). Black bears climb trees, but are likely to run away, not chase you up.

Should the bear charge, lie down and play dead. Roll up in a ball with hands over your neck to protect it. It will be hard, but don't move or scream. Though the bear may swat at you, it will lose interest if you are still. Do not move until the bear is far away as it may attack again if it detects movement or sound.

To prevent chance meetings in the first place, never set up camp in an area that has bear prints, bear scat, or animal carcasses. Always hang food at least 10 feet (3 m) up a tree and 5 feet (1.5 m) away from the trunk. Keep a clean camp and get rid of garbage daily. Wash utensils after use. Make noise while walking — sing or talk so that you don't startle bears.

If a bear is trying to get into your house, make loud noises to drive them away. Never corner a wild animal, and give them plenty of space to escape.

BULL CHARGE

If you suddenly find yourself in a bull's territory and he begins to charge, drop any object you may be carrying in their path. Bulls will often stop to investigate, which will give you time to escape. If the bull starts after you again, keep removing clothing items, keep dropping them, and keep running.

CAR ACCIDENTS

In case of an impending accident, don't panic — keep your head and steer to do the minimum amount of damage. Make sure your seat belt is tightly fastened. If the brakes fail, shift the engine into a lower gear and use the hand brake.

Once the accident has occurred, switch off the vehicle but leave the key in the ignition. Set the parking brake and turn the flashers on. Watch out for other cars, get out of your vehicle, and drop flares to warn traffic approaching from behind. If you don't have flares, ask someone to warn traffic.

Do not allow cigarette smoking near the vehicle. Treat injured persons as necessary, but do not move seriously injured persons unless they are in immediate danger. Cover victims lightly with a blanket and reassure them that help is on the way.

If a car crashes into water, it will stay afloat longer if the windows are closed. Switch on all the lights. Keep a hand on the door handles. When water level is chin-deep, open the door, take a deep breath, and swim for the surface. If there are multiple people in the car, link arms and make a human chain until everyone is out so that the door remains open and no one is trapped.

Whenever your car breaks down, turn off the engine, lights, and radio to conserve the charge in the battery. Lift the hood (a common distress signal) and tie a bright colored cloth to the antenna to signal that help is needed. Keep car doors locked and roll up the windows. If someone comes to the car, send them for help without opening the door or window.

If your car fails in cold country, car upholstery can be cut and stuffed into your clothing for insulation. Park in a protected place with southeastern or eastern exposure if you can.

In all cases of car breakdown, stay with your car, as it can be used as a shelter.

CHILDBIRTH

If medical care is far away and birth is imminent, you may need to be prepared to do it yourself. These instructions are only for those times when a qualified medical practitioner or midwife is unavailable — in other words, an emergency situation! In all such cases, have the mother and child pay a visit to a health-care provider as soon as possible after the birth.

First, find a clean, warm place for the birth to occur. If you'll be delivering the baby, wash your hands and scrub your nails. Shake them dry rather than using a towel. (*Note:* Keep any open cuts or wounds away from the mother and baby. If available, wear latex gloves.)

Have the mother take a warm shower, if possible, to help keep the process clean and help her to relax. A bath is also an option, as long as the mother's water hasn't burst. Pull clean socks and a shirt on the mother, then prepare the bed. Put on a clean fitted sheet, then a plastic sheet, then another fitted sheet so that after the birth, fresh, clean bedding will be ready.

For tying off the umbilical cord, cut three lengths of a clean material — cotton sheet, shoelaces, cord, or whatever is available — each about 9 inches (23 cm) long. If possible, sterilize some scissors and the three lengths of material by boiling them in water for twenty minutes, then wrapping in a clean cloth. Avoid touching anything you have sterilized until you need to use it.

Have a sanitary napkin ready for the mother after the placenta is delivered.

Make the About-to-Be Mom More Comfortable

Walking, standing, and squatting will help shorten labor. A 1,000-mg calcium and 500-mg magnesium supplement taken at the beginning may raise the mother's threshold for pain. Four pellets of homeopathic *Arnica* dissolved under the tongue may help ease the pain.

Encourage the mother to urinate frequently; put a portable potty or bowl by the bed if necessary. For strength, offer a cup of raspberry leaf or ginger tea with honey.

Encourage the mother to breathe deeply in and out with each contraction. She should do her best to relax and even sleep between contractions. Massaging the lower back can help relieve back pain.

The mother should not push while her contractions are more than two minutes apart. As labor progresses, she will then feel a powerful urge to bear down. Encourage her. Apply cloths that have been soaked in warm ginger tea or water to the area around the vaginal opening to help the skin stretch.

Lavender essential oil is great to have at delivery time. The mother will likely be doing lots of deep breathing and will be energized and uplifted by the smells of this essential oil occasionally being wafted under her nose.

Delivering the Goods

Squatting during delivery can help decrease pushing time, lower the rate of cesareans, and reduce the need for forceps. That said, allow the mother to get into any position that feels comfortable.

Encourage the mother to go limp like a rag doll while breathing deeply as this will help her to open. She should not hold her breath or push down during delivery contractions. Panting, short breaths with the mouth open helps the baby to be born slowly with less risk of tearing.

Support the baby's head as it emerges. If there is a membrane over the baby's face, remove it immediately but gently. Break it with your fingernails right below the baby's nose where it is less tight so the baby won't inhale the fluids.

Support the baby's shoulders as they emerge, but avoid pulling. If the umbilical cord is wrapped around the baby's neck, hook your finger around the cord and loop it over the baby's head. (*Note:* Should the baby's bottom or feet emerge first, support but don't pull the baby.)

Once the shoulders have emerged, use your hands to support and ease the baby's body slightly up so the mouth has more breathing room. Gently raising the baby's head will help the second shoulder to emerge. It is not unusual for the baby to slip back a bit between contractions.

Encourage the mother to continue taking panting breaths to prevent the baby from coming out too quickly. After the shoulders are out, the rest of the body should soon follow. The baby is likely to be very slippery so be careful!

Helping the Baby

If the baby isn't breathing right away use an infant-sized, sterilized bulb syringe to help. Squeeze the bulb, then place the tip of the syringe into the baby's mouth. Quickly move the tip around in the mouth, while slowly allowing the bulb to take in air and suck out mucus. You can also use the syringe to suck mucus out of the nostrils. Stroking the baby's throat from the bottom of the neck to the chin with the side of your index finger can further clear mucus.

Rub the baby's feet and back or flick the bottoms of the feet with your index finger. Speak gently to the baby, letting him know how glad you are that he is here and that he is loved.

Do not spank the baby's bottom. If the baby doesn't start breathing within a few seconds of birth, elevate his neck and tilt the head back slightly to open air passages. Open your mouth and seal it over the baby's nose and mouth and *gently* blow a puff of air into the baby's mouth. Blow at a rate of twenty puffs a minute. Stop as soon as the baby's chest starts to rise and fall on its own.

If the baby's breathing is fine and the cord is long enough, place the baby on the mother's chest. Put his head slightly lower than his feet to help clear any additional mucus.

When the baby has been delivered, it will be covered with a creamy white coating called the vernix, which is rich in nutrients. Don't wash it off, except around the nose and mouth. Instead, allow it to be absorbed, as it helps to protect the baby's skin.

Encourage the mother to offer the baby her breast. If the baby starts to nurse, it will help the uterus contract and expel the placenta.

Wait until the umbilical cord has stopped pulsing before cutting it as the baby is still receiving oxygen and nutrients through the cord. When the cord is no longer pulsing, tie it closed with the sterilized cloth, shoelace, or cord about 6 inches (15 cm) from the baby's belly. Tie a second cloth strip around the umbilical cord eight inches (20 cm) from the baby's belly. Make sure the knots are tight enough to prevent blood leakage but not so tight they cut into the cord. Cut through the umbilical cord in between the two knots with either sterilized scissors or a clean, unused razor blade.

Cord Care

Squeeze a bit of breast milk into the baby's navel area every couple of hours as breast milk contains natural antibodies. Powdered goldenseal or rosemary can also be sprinkled on the area at each diaper change. If inflammation occurs, also apply a few drops of calendula or echinacea tincture. The cord should be kept dry and outside the diaper.

Care After Birth

Place a bowl between the mother's legs to catch the placenta. If the placenta hasn't come within two hours of birth, help the mother to squat, as squatting may ease delivery. Do not pull on the umbilical cord to hasten the placenta's delivery. The placenta should be examined by a midwife or doctor — she will be able to tell if the whole thing has been delivered. If there is any hemorrhaging, put both hands, one on top of the other, on the abdomen below the mother's navel and lean down on the area. Continue pressing until the bleeding stops.

Clean the mother and place a sanitary napkin or clean cloth over the vaginal opening. Offer the mother something to eat and drink. For the first hour after birth keep a close watch on the mother and massage the stomach above the uterus firmly, until it feels like a fist.

A good tea to give after birth is shepherd's purse, to minimize any bleeding. A woman shouldn't lose more than 2 cups (460 ml) of blood during the birthing process. If bleeding is excessive, stir ¼ teaspoon

(1 ml) cayenne pepper into a glass of warm water sweetened with honey and lemon or give 1 dropperful of cayenne pepper, nettle, or shepherd's purse tincture every ten minutes. Massaging the lower abdomen in a firm but gentle circular motion will help the uterus to become harder and decrease bleeding.

As for the baby, keep him or her warm. Cover the head and body to conserve heat loss, and put the baby by his or her mother. Putting the baby on his or her side will allow mucus to drain.

Ideally the mother should rest for at least five days following the birth.

While all births not monitored by a midwife or obstetrician should be followed up by a visit to your health-care professional, be sure to seek immediate medical attention if:

- The mother knows she has a serious health condition or is prone to seizures
- There is excessive bleeding before the birth

MAINTAINING A PREGNANCY

About one in ten pregnancies ends in miscarriage. Seventy-five percent of the miscarriages occur within the first twelve weeks. Many occur before a woman even realizes she is pregnant. Environmental pollutants, drugs, stress, overexposure to radiation, fibroid tumors, infection, structural abnormalities, fetal abnormalities, and nutritional deficiencies can all be contributing factors to miscarriage.

Miscarriage is sometimes nature's way of letting go of a being that may be less than perfect. This is something important to consider before trying to halt a miscarriage.

It is only during the first stage, referred to as a threatened miscarriage, that you can prevent the end of a pregnancy. Bleeding, spotting, and cramping are all symptoms. When the blood becomes heavy and bright red, doctors feel it's too late to prevent a miscarriage.

If a miscarriage threatens and medical assistance is not available, lie down and elevate your feet for 24 hours.

Black haw is a powerful uterine sedative. It also strengthens a weak cervix, and has helped many women continue a pregnancy. In case of a threatened miscarriage, take 1 dropperful of black haw tincture every 2 hours (waking hours — discontinue while sleeping) for 2–3 days.

- Labor takes longer than 48 hours (or doesn't seem to be progressing)
- There are feces in the baby's nose or mouth
- Bleeding is excessive after the birth
- The mother manifests signs of shock
- The mother becomes unconscious
- The mother has chills and fever
- The placenta takes longer than two hours to be delivered
- The placenta is not whole or is delivered in pieces
- The baby did not present head first

COLD (severe)

(See also *Hypothermia* on page 66, *Frostbite* on page 58, and *Making a Fire* on page 104)

Severe cold, whether out in the wilderness or in your home when the power has failed, can quickly lead to a life-threatening situation. The first thing to do, of course, is don several layers of dry clothing, and a hat to conserve body heat. (We lose about 50 percent of our body heat through the head and neck.) Depending on where you are and what supplies are available to you, there are several additional things you can do to avoid frostbite, hypothermia, and other cold-induced, life-threatening situations:

- When exposed to severe cold, wrinkle your face and exercise your hands to keep blood circulating in those easily frostbitten areas.
- If you're with a group of people, huddle together. Take turns putting different people in the middle (the warmest position). Toes and feet can be rewarmed by placing them on the belly of a friend.
- Avoid contact with cold, metal objects (remove any metal jewelry), as well as cold foods, water, and wind. Wading through very cold water can be fatal.
- Ditch the cigarettes — they'll constrict your already cold-constricted blood vessels.
- Don't drink alcohol — it will lower your body temperature.
- Sprinkle a bit of cayenne pepper between your shoes and socks to keep your feet warm. An extra pair of socks can be used as mittens to keep your hands warm. (Remember, mittens are warmer than gloves.)

- Stuff clothes with dry grass, moss, leaves, or crumpled newspaper to provide insulation.
- Replace wet clothing with dry whenever possible. If clothes become damp while you're camping overnight, spread them between a sleeping bag liner and the bag itself. Or spread them beneath the sleeping bag and sleep on top of them.
- If there's snow around and you've accidentally gotten wet, rolling around in the fluffy snow will blot up much of the moisture.

EARTHQUAKE

If you feel the earth rumbling under your feet, get under something heavy to avoid being hit by falling objects. If indoors, take shelter under a sturdy table or other heavy furniture object. Standing under a door frame can offer protection as it is usually the strongest part of a building. An inside corner of the house can also offer protection. Do not run outdoors as you may be hit by falling debris. Stay away from glass objects, mirrors, and windows.

If you are outside, stay there. If on a hill, watch for rock slides — getting to the top is safest. Keep away from tall buildings, trees, power lines, and any other collapsible object. Cover your head as much as possible. If the earthquake is strong enough to cause you to lose your balance, lie flat on the ground. Stay out of basements, subways, or tunnels, which could become blocked.

If you're in a car, stop and stay put. Dive for the floor and crouch below the seat level if possible.

When the earthquake has stopped, watch out for fallen cables, broken roads, and damaged buildings and bridges that could collapse. Aftershocks may follow.

If your house seems okay, enter carefully (if outside during the quake) and check for fire, gas leaks, and water leaks. Don't smoke or light a match. Use only a flashlight. Turn off gas, water, and electricity if you suspect any hazard or are advised to do so by local authorities.

If your house is damaged, consider building a shelter from available debris. Some experts feel it's safer to stay in a temporary shelter than to return to a damaged building.

FIRE

Depending on the circumstance, fire can both put you in grave danger, or save your life. Whether trapped in a burning building or huddled over a small flame on a cold night, it's important to know fire's habits and how to control it. Read on.

When Your Clothing Is on Fire

"Stop! Drop! Roll!" is the emergency adage that can save your life. It's the fastest way to smother the flames.

If you see someone running from a fire wearing burning clothes, stop the person and throw him or her to the ground, burning side up. Beat the flames downward, away from the head. Use water to douse the flames or smother the fire with a blanket, rug, coat, or drapes, but only after the person is on the ground. If water is unavailable, liquids such as milk may be used, but never spirits such as gin or whiskey. Avoid using a fire extinguisher as it contains chemicals.

After the fire is out do not try to remove clothing stuck on the skin. Get medical assistance and treat for shock (see page 77) or burns (see page 39). Remove any smoldering clothing and any jewelry or tight clothes around the area of burns as swelling may occur. Protect yourself — smoldering clothes can be hotter than the fire itself. Submerge any small burned areas in cold slow running water for at least ten minutes. Do not apply water to deep or widespread burns.

Forest Fire

If you're trapped in a forest fire, your greatest danger is suffocation. Cup your hands over your nose and mouth to help cool down hot air and fend off sparks that can damage the respiratory system. Cover your head and body with a wet coat or blanket to protect your skin, and avoid dry vegetation, which can easily ignite.

Forest fires burn more quickly uphill than downhill; they can travel uphill faster than a person can run. If you're ever trapped uphill from flames, search for the largest open area possible and stay in the middle of it.

If on foot, get low when flames are close. Jump into a body of water if possible, or a gully or ravine if you can find one. If you need to run through stands of trees choose hardwoods rather than softwoods, as softwoods burn more rapidly. It is best to run through areas where there is little vegetation or run through an area that has already burned. Be on the lookout for falling branches and flying embers.

If the fire's coming your way and there's no avoiding it, dig a hole for yourself in the ground, get in, and cover yourself with earth. People have survived fires by burying themselves in dirt and allowing the fire to burn on over them. Hold your breath as much as possible as the fire leaps over you if you're in a gully or hole in the ground to avoid burning your lungs.

Making a Fire

Fire can keep dangerous animals away. Its smoke can repel insects, and its flames provide warmth and cook food. However, fire uses up nature's resources, and campfires are a common cause of forest fires, so it is best to build one only if it's really needed.

To make a fire, you need a safe burning area, a spark, tinder, small kindling, and larger pieces of wood or other fuel.

Site. To prepare an area for a fire, first clear away any surrounding brush. Dig a small fire pit or build a small circle of stones to contain the coals and ashes. When at a campsite where a fire pit already exists, use it rather than cause another burned spot in the camp area. Always have something handy to put the fire out if necessary.

Spark. Matches are the easiest tool for sparking a fire. They should be stored in several waterproof containers and distributed throughout your supplies. That way, if you lose some of your pack you'll still have some matches available.

You can also spark a fire with a flashlight battery and a small, thin piece of wire. Remove the wire's insulation and, using a piece of wood or insulation to avoid getting burned, hold each end of the wire to an end of the battery. The wire will soon heat up. Hold the wire against some tinder and blow till it catches fire.

You can also start a fire by focusing the sun's rays onto a small pile of tinder with a magnifying glass or lens from a telescope or binoculars. And don't forget the cigarette lighter in the car as a fire-starting source.

Tinder. Tinder must be dry to ignite. Fire burns upward, so if you want the tinder to ignite, place it on top of the spark, rather than on the sides. Good sources of tinder include birch bark strips; abandoned bird's nests; cedar bark; dry grass; dry moss; lichen; dead evergreen needles; feathers; pussy willow fuzz; dried puffball mushrooms; elder pith; down from cattail, milkweed, fireweed, and goldenrod; paper; resinous pine knots; straw; leaves; even shredded clothing fragments, cotton, or bandages from a first-aid kit. Dried pitch scraped from the outside of spruce, pine, or other conifers provides a powder that burns easily. If everything is wet, look for tinder at the base of trees or underneath rock overhangs.

Kindling. Good sources of kindling include dry twigs from wood that burns fast and hot, such as alder, cedar, hemlock, pine, and willow. Softwood twigs flare quickly and are especially good.

Wood. The ideal wood for a controlled, warming fire is slow and even burning. Good choices include beech, hickory, and oak. Middling choices include birch, fir, and maple. Standing deadwood is ideal for burning as fallen wood will have collected lots of moisture. Damp wood, however, produces lots of smoke, which may be desirable if you want to drive off insects. Should you be without an ax, stouter branches or rotten logs can be broken by smashing them over a rock. Dried cattle or other animal dung, tumbleweed, and driftwood all are potential fuels.

Fire-building. Prepare the fire pit, then make a base of tinder and a teepee shape of kindling around it. Light the tinder. Blow gently as the tinder glows, adding more kindling in small amounts. As the kindling catches fire, add larger twigs. Add branches loosely so that there is adequate air circulation. Never add gasoline to get a fire going as this can cause an explosion. Should a fire appear to go out during the night, clearing away some ashes may expose some hot coals still glowing that can be used to rebuild the fire. It is important to remember these coals when you leave your campsite: Make sure the fire is *completely* extinguished.

FLOOD

When preparing your home for a flood, place sandbags along the outside thresholds of doors to reduce water invasion. Seal up the central heating flue and other ventilation ducts. Tape up windows if flooding is likely to be heavy and seal off both exterior and interior doors with blankets, old carpet, or whatever else is available. Have something to signal with, such as a bright cloth. Turn off the gas and electricity. Gather emergency food supplies, drinking water in well-sealed containers, candles, waterproof matches, and warm clothes. Bring movable objects and outdoor furniture inside to reduce floating debris.

If you're trapped indoors by a flood, go to the top floor, taking with you anything that will float: wood, foam mattresses, spare tires, and the like. If possible, move your valuables up, too. Should you be relegated to the roof, set up a shelter. If it's a sloping roof, tie everyone to a structure, such as the chimney. Be on the alert for floating snakes and other animals, as well as boards with nails and other dangerous objects. Keep a flotation device with you. Remain where you are until the water stops rising.

People have survived floods by tying themselves into a tree. Should water rise this high, be prepared to build a raft using anything that can float, and any sheets or ropes that are available to tie things together.

Food touched by floodwaters is deemed contaminated. Treat all drinking water before consuming. (See *Water Shortage,* page 114.)

ICE RESCUE

If someone is stuck out on thin ice, or has fallen through thin ice into the cold waters below, do not follow them out there in a rescue attempt! In order to help them, you need to stay on the shore or on solid ice — you won't be any use to the person if you fall through as well. Instead, reach out to them from a safe location with a long, sturdy, lightweight tool — a light ladder is ideal. For even greater reach, you can tie a strong line to its lowest rung and slide the ladder out toward him or her. Ropes, buoys, and poles can all be used. You can even use a chain of people, provided they all lie on their stomachs to disperse their weight over the ice. Even after the person has been dragged to safety, the rescue may not be over. He or she may have inhaled water, or may be suffering from hypothermia. Refer to Drowning, on page 49, or Hypothermia, on page 66.

LIGHTNING

Lightning kills about three hundred people in the United States each year and seriously injures twice that many. It does not have to strike a person directly in order to kill. It can strike a long way from the storm with which it's associated.

If you get caught in an electrical storm, avoid moist areas, tall trees, lone boulders, and overhangs. If you are near a lone tree, boulder, or tall building, move away quickly as they can become channels for the lightning. If you're at the mouth of a cave, get deeper into the cave. If you have to seek shelter among trees, do so in a large stand and crouch as low as possible. If you're on top of a mountain, head for lower, level ground and kneel down.

Stay away from metal objects such as fences, golf clubs, and umbrellas. Be wary of bridges. Remove any metallic objects you may be wearing.

If your skin starts tingling and your hair stands on end, lightning may be about to strike where you're standing. If out in the open, drop to the ground and lie flat to lessen your risk of being struck immediately. If you're near a tall object and you can't get away, kneel down, keeping your feet and knees close together on something dry like a piece of wood. Keep your feet off the ground and on the dry material. Bend over and keep your head to your knees, drawing in all your extremities so that very little of your body is in contact with the ground. Avoid placing your hands on the ground.

If you're swimming or in a boat when an electrical storm blows in, immediately get to shore. Water conducts electricity and lightning can "spatter" when it hits something in the water — it disperses over a wide area upon impact. If you're caught in a large boat and you can't get to shore, go below deck. The helmsperson may need to stay at his or her post, but he or she should avoid touching anything metal.

If you're in a car when the storm hits, park safely, close the windows, and stay put. The wheels provide insulation from electrical charges.

Once you find shelter, stay indoors until the storm is over. If you're in a house or other building, stay away from open doors and windows, metal pipes, and electric conductors such as sinks and stoves. Unplug or refrain from using electric appliances. Lightning can enter through phone wires so it is best not to use a telephone. It is generally considered safe to be inside a building, but isolated barns and sheds are a higher risk.

LOST IN THE WILDERNESS

If you're lost in the wilderness, the most important thing to do is to keep your head and not panic. Check your map and consider the terrain you've just passed through. To help get your bearings, look at the vegetation around you. Depending on where you are, any of the following could work as nature's directional tips:

- Most trees tend to lean to the east unless there are prevailing wind factors. Exception: Alders, poplars, and willows tend to lean to the south.
- Hemlocks, pines, and spruces are bushiest on their south side.
- Age rings in a stump are usually widest on the south side.
- Ant hills tend to be on the south side of trees and objects.
- Vegetation tends to be larger on northern slopes and smaller and denser on southern slopes.
- Moss (not lichens) will usually be found growing on the north side of tree trunks, especially if the tree is out in the open and is exposed to sunlight.
- As the sun sets in the west, north is on the right side of the sun.
- Woodpeckers tend to peck into the east side of trees.

If you are lost, it's best to stay where you are — search teams will find it easier to gauge the area where you might be if you don't move around too much. If you do move, look for something that indicates the presence of people — a road, building, or power line. If you're with friends, don't split up. Take turns hollering or blowing a whistle. Leave signs of your route — deliberate footprints, bent branches, bits of fabric. If lost in a forested area, stay in the openings to make it easier for rescue aircraft to spot you. The sign recognized for distress is three whistles, gunshots, or light flashes.

Walk downhill in a straight line. Keep streams within earshot, but don't walk right next to them. Following them too closely could lead into dangerously deep ravines. Follow a watercourse downstream as this is more likely to lead to a populated area. Once on level ground there may be animal trails beside the water, which will be easy to follow. Should you find a road, it's wise to follow it, even if it isn't the right road.

When it gets dark, stay put and light a fire if possible (see Making a Fire on page 104). Traveling at night is not recommended as you can encounter too many hazards. It is ideal to set up camp an hour before nightfall. (**Note:** If you happen to be lost in the desert, the opposite is true — do your traveling at night, when it's cool, and find a spot with some shade for resting during the day.)

Be Prepared

Always venture into a wilderness area with waterproof outer clothing, some food, water, a hat, gloves, a map and compass, waterproof matches or lighter, whistle, flashlight, first-aid kit, paper and pencil, and a large plastic trash bag, which can serve as a rain poncho or mini-tent.

Check weather reports before leaving. Always tell someone where you are going and when you expect to return. If you're exploring from a campsite, leave a note detailing your plans and who is in your party. Then, as you move, keep track of where you are with a map, pencil, and compass. Or draw a map as you go, indicating significant landmarks.

Foraging for Food

In case you're ever stuck in the woods without supplies, don't worry about your next meal. You're surrounded by edible plants.

Acorns can be shelled and soaked in running stream water for twenty-four hours to leach out bitter tannins, then ground into meal. They can also be boiled in several changes of water or roasted as a coffee substitute.

Cattails are one of the best wild-food plants. Flour can be made from peeled, dried roots. The new, white sprouts can be eaten raw or cooked. Young shoots are peeled and cooked as a vegetable. Pollen spikes must be cooked, and then can be eaten like corn on the cob.

Dandelions are versatile. Young leaves can be eaten in salads; blossoms can be cooked or eaten raw. If older leaves are used, boil in two changes of water to remove the bitter principles. Roots can be cleaned and cooked like carrots. Roasted roots are used as a coffee substitute.

Lamb's-quarters are packed with iron and beta carotene. Eat raw in salads. Cook like spinach. Seeds can be ground into a flour. Can be fed to animals as fodder.

Mustard plants can add spice to your diet. The greens can be cooked and the flowers eaten raw. Young leaves may be finely chopped and added to salads. Older leaves can be cooked as a green vegetable. Flowers are edible.

Pine nuts, though small, are a delicacy. They can be harvested from the insides of pine cones.

Seaweeds are full of minerals and fiber, and most are edible. Collect only those growing, not what washes up on shore. Reject any that smell bad or cause skin irritation when crushed with the fingers. Rinse in fresh water if possible. Seaweed can be dried for later use, but if remoistened will quickly decay.

Trees that have edible inner barks, buds, and shoots (usually best in spring and eaten raw) include aspens and poplars (*Populus* spp.), linden (*Tilia americana*), birch (*Betula* spp.), maple (*Acer* spp.), spruce (*Picea* spp.), and willow (*Salix* spp.).

EATING IN THE WILD

Do not eat unfamiliar wild foods unless it's an absolute emergency. Better yet, as part of your preparation process, buy a good wild foods identification book and practice some wild food cookery as part of your regular diet.

Do not count on the fact that because a bird or animal eats a food that humans can also eat it. Avoid mushrooms altogether unless you are already an expert. Avoid plants with milky sap.

If you're in a group, one person at a time should test a potential food plant. First rub some of the plant's juices on a tender part of the body, such as the inside of the elbow or under the arm. If swelling, redness, or irritation occurs, don't eat that one. Rub a bit of a crushed plant around the inside of the lower lip. Place a smaller than fingernail-size piece on the tip of the tongue and wait five minutes. If any burning or swelling occurs discard the plant. If no signs of toxicity have occurred, take a larger piece of the plant (about 2 inches or 5 cm), chew and swallow. Wait two hours. Be on the alert for nausea or diarrhea. If either occurs, eat no more. If all seems okay, repeat the process with a larger portion of the plant, about six inches (15 cm). If no ill effects are noticed, the plant is probably safe to eat.

While you are testing a potential new food, avoid eating anything else. Boiling the food in two changes of water will make it even safer to eat. As time goes by, try this with more plants to increase the variety of your diet.

And don't worry about getting enough to eat: The average person can survive for three weeks without food.

MOUNTAIN LION

If you come face to face with a mountain lion do not turn and run or you will provoke an attack. Face the cat and speak in a normal voice. If that doesn't make it leave, wave your arms and start yelling. Throwing something at the cat may or may not work — it could either make the cat run or attack.

In mountain lion country, be careful when going around bends and under overhangs — make some noise so that you don't take a cat by surprise. Stay in a group or at least have another person with you. Should you see tracks and scat, make noise, talk loudly, and sing or play music.

PORCUPINE

In a porcupine-human encounter, porcupines will do their best to escape, so give them plenty of room. Should you get quills stuck in you, soak the wounds in vinegar to soften the quills and gently pull them out. Seek medical attention if you cannot remove the quills or the site becomes infected.

QUICKSAND

Bogs and quicksand can be fatal to an unsuspecting hiker. Avoid depressions where light, spikey, green grass tufts are growing; they can indicate a swamp or bog.

If you do fall into a patch of quicksand, first try running or jumping to solid ground. The next best approach is to fall to your knees and get to shore by grabbing on to grass or roots to propel yourself to safety. Spread out your body weight as widely as possible and move slowly and deliberately. Quick movements will create pockets that will cause you to sink more rapidly. Discard any pack or items that will weigh you down.

If you find yourself stuck, fall gently onto your back with your arms spread wide. If you are by yourself, stay on your back and use backstroke movements to get to firmer ground. Be patient, move slowly. Even if it takes an hour to move just a few feet, this position is your best way to survive.

If someone is with you, have them pull you out with a rope, stick, or other means.

RABIES

Rabies is a virus that can be transmitted through a scratch, bite, or lick from a warm-blooded, infected animal. Bats, cows, dogs, foxes, skunks, raccoons, and in rare cases rabbits and rats are all known to carry the virus.

Other potential carriers are cats, deer, horses, weasels, and wolves. Because responsible owners usually vaccinate their dogs against rabies, less than one hundred dogs are proven to have rabies in the United States each year.

Rabid animals may appear sick and overly friendly. If you are bitten, capture the animal if possible (with great care) and have it observed for ten days for signs of drooling, foaming from the mouth, and nervousness. If it is necessary to kill the animal, leave it whole and keep it refrigerated or packed in ice until you can bring it to be tested. Rabies can be identified by a lab technician when he or she examines the brain of the killed animal. Should it be impossible to either catch the animal or kill it, give a report of the animal's appearance and last-sighted location to law enforcement personnel.

Symptoms of rabies include intense thirst, headache, and muscle spasms. They can take as long as ten weeks from the time of infection to appear, and by then the disease is often fatal. Treatment involves a series of five shots in the arm or buttocks — and a tetanus booster for good measure. This treatment is recommended for all potential rabies cases.

RADIATION

Radiation exposure from a large-scale disaster at a nuclear power plant or weapons facility or from a nuclear bomb can cause weakness, nausea, and vomiting as well as cancer, birth defects, and death.

If such a disaster strikes your area, listen to the radio for warnings to evacuate. Get underground into a cellar if possible. If you can't, middle or ground floors of buildings are safer than top floors. Choose rooms with the least number of outside walls. Stock food, water, and hygiene supplies. Buffer walls, doors, and windows with anything available — brick, hardpacked earth, sandbags, and so forth. Shut off the water main so that contaminated water does not enter your area. Even boiled water that has been exposed to radiation will not be safe for consumption. Have a fire extinguisher handy. Cover exposed skin with anything available.

After you've been exposed, wash your entire body with clean water. If pure water is not available, and you are in a shelter with an earthen floor, rub soil on your body and clothing, then throw it out. Cover your nose, eyes, and mouth with a damp cloth to prevent contact between radioactive particles and your mucous membranes.

In a radiation-contaminated zone, stay in the protected, indoor shelter you've created for as long as possible. Venture outdoors only when absolutely necessary. For the first two weeks, limit any necessary outdoor time to no more than half an hour a day. After that, limit your outdoor time to the shortest periods possible. Remove your outer clothing before reentering your shelter. Wash all clothing and skin exposed to the outside air, and apply any healing herbal salve to any skin ulcerations that develop.

Avoid water from exposed sources. Roots and underground growing things will be safer to eat than aboveground plants. Look for foods with removable coverings: nuts in shells, eggs, vegetables that can be peeled, and vegetables that are protected by outer leaves. Animals that are outside will be contaminated so don't think of hunting them. Wipe off any containers of food before opening. Take 9 250-mg kelp tablets daily to help minimize radioactive levels in the body. Eat miso soup and seaweed daily. If there's pure water available, soak in a bathtub to which 1 pound (454 g) each of sea salt and baking soda have been added. To soothe internal irritation as a result of radiation exposure, drink aloe vera juice — 1 ounce (29 ml) 3 times daily. Aloe vera gel can also be applied to radiation burns. Use chlorophyll as a supplement to aid in detoxifying. Eat plenty of pectin-rich foods, such as apples and carrots, as they will bind with toxins and help flush them out of the body.

TORNADO

In tornado-prone areas, know in advance where you might go should a tornado strike. If you have ample warning, bring loose furniture, garden tools, and planters inside as they can become dangerous when airborne.

When a tornado is approaching, get into a basement, storm cellar, or the most solid structure possible. Stay away from windows. If you can't get below ground, take refuge in a small bathroom or closet in a central part of the house away from doors and windows. Wrap yourself in blankets or overcoats as protection against flying debris. Get under a heavy object if available. If in a commercial building, the hallway may be the safest. If in bed when the tornado strikes, get under the bed. If in a mobile home, get into a more secure shelter if possible.

If you're on the road, remember that tornadoes change directions and may be difficult to outrun in a car. Get out and take shelter in a building, or get to a highway overpass and go under it for cover.

In the open, get into a ditch or any depression in the ground and lie on your stomach; protect your head with your arms.

WATER SHORTAGE

If you hear of an impending disaster that may affect your water supply, immediately fill bathtubs, sinks, and clean bottles. If the water supply to homes and buildings has already been shut off or disrupted, the pipes in your home may still contain water. Beginning at the top floor and working down, drain water in the pipes into containers. Keep the faucets open to provide air vent. When you reach the lowest floor, shut off the hot-water heater, then drain it as needed. Although bacteria in the pipes is usually not substantial, water taken from pipes should still be purified.

Rainwater can be collected from rain spouts and diverted into clean containers. Also collect rainwater by setting cups or containers under branches and ledges. Cloths can also be spread out to collect water.

How to Purify Water

Failure to purify water can cause parasitic invasion, misery, and in some cases death. Yet three drops of iodine tincture will purify 1 quart (920 ml) of water in ten minutes. Clorox can also be used as a water purifier — it contains chlorine — four drops per quart (920 ml) or ten drops per gallon (3.8 l). If the water is very dirty or you are storing it, double the amount of iodine or Clorox. If the water to which you've added Clorox is very cold, let stand twenty minutes before drinking. Water can be stored indefinitely in gallon jugs if ½ tablespoon (7.5 ml) Clorox is added.

Boiling water is safer than chemical purification. Purify by boiling 5 minutes (plus 1 minute more for every 1,000 feet [300 m] above sea level). To improve the taste of boiled — or stored — water, pour it from one container to another to oxygenate it.

If nothing else is available, place water in clean glass and allow to cook in the sun for 12 hours to help sterilize it. While this will help, it's not a guaranteed method for sterilization.

How to Find Fresh Water

Water seeks the lowest levels, so look in valley bottoms where water naturally drains. Look for areas of prolific vegetation. Birds tend to fly over water in areas where it is scarce. Birds flying low and straight — particularly at dawn or dusk — are usually headed toward water. Should you find a watering hole, however, with no plant life thriving around it, use caution as this may indicate it's contaminated in some way. In desert areas, look for a dry lakebed and start digging at the lowest point.

Look for rain trapped in plant leaves. Collect dew early in the morning with a sponge or tie cloths to your ankles and stomp around. Then wring or suck the water out. Windows of homes and cars as well as other cold and metal surfaces will collect dew. Dew is as clean as rainwater, although in cities it can be polluted. Avoid collecting dew from areas that have been sprayed with pesticides or herbicides. Sponges and clothes left on greenery overnight might collect enough moisture for you to have a sponge bath the following morning.

Trees can also be a source of moisture. The sap from birch and maple trees can be drunk. Cut a V-shaped gash in the trunk and insert spouts made from hollow elder limbs at low angles.

Unpleasant-tasting water can be sweetened by boiling it with a piece of hardwood charcoal for 15 minutes. Strain or allow the water to settle.

A water still can be created by digging a hole 3 feet (1 m) deep and 4 feet (1.2 m) wide. Place a container in the bottom along with a length of plastic tubing that reaches the top of the hole. Anchor the tube to the top edge of the hole. Cover the hole with a plastic sheet that is weighed down in the middle, forming a cone a

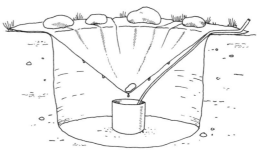

Water stills are a traditional, time-tested method for gathering water.

few inches above the collecting receptacle. The sun's heat will warm the soil and cause the evaporation of moisture, which will collect on the underside of the plastic and trickle down to the point of the cone, where it will fall into the container. You can make several of these stills. This water does not need to be treated. You can suck water through the tube to avoid disturbing the still. Try to position the still where the sun will be hot and the soil moist by selecting areas with green vegetation. Adding nonpoisonous plants to the pit will increase the amount of water collected. Move the still to another area every few days.

In colder regions, keep in mind that snow must be melted before it is eaten to avoid digestive distress, and eating ice can injure the mouth and cause further dehydration. Ice requires 50 percent less fuel to melt than snow, and lower layers of snow will produce more water than upper layers. Use a dark colored container to melt snow or ice. Cold does not kill germs, so ice should be treated before drinking.

Saltwater is unfit to drink. It's a laxative, which will leave you dehydrated. Old sea ice that is bluish gray is not salty — taste before melting.

HOW TO AVOID DEHYDRATION WHEN WATER IS SCARCE

The average person can survive for three days without water. Most people need at least 1 quart (920 ml) of drinking water daily, although 3 quarts (2700 ml) is preferable. To reduce the risk of dehydration when water is scarce, follow these common-sense tips:

- **When drinking, moisten the lips, tongue, and throat before swallowing.** Gulping too much too fast can cause vomiting.
- **Don't ration water.** Use what you need today and find more tomorrow. Suck on a pebble, button, or other small object to help alleviate thirst.
- **Avoid alcohol and smoking.** Both are dehydrating.
- **Breathe through the nose.**
- **Stay in the shade.**
- **Minimize activity.** Rest and sleep are the best way to conserve fluids when water is scarce. Minimize conversation as well — talking can be dehydrating.

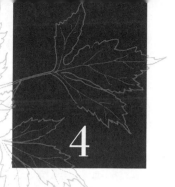

STOCKING A FIRST-AID KIT

K eep all your first-aid kits out of reach of children. Make sure every-thing is well labeled and has directions, such as "for external use only." Date substances that have a limited shelf life. Store your kit in a cool, dry place.

AN HERBAL FIRST-AID KIT

Your mother falls down the stairs. Your toddler scrapes his knee. Your sister comes down with food poisoning. Your husband gets frostbite. To treat any and all of the injuries and conditions resulting from these common events, you need a first-aid kit that can handle just about any-thing. Most of these items are readily available in pharmacies and health food stores. Here's what the kit should include:

Ace bandage. To wrap sprains, and apply pressure to bleeding wounds.

Adhesive dressings, butterfly bandages, gauze pads, roll of adhesive tape. In an emergency situation, you can use a clean plantain leaf taped over a wound as a bandage.

Alcohol. To sterilize tweezers, needles.

Analgesic balm. To alleviate pain. Apply topically.

Arnica oil. For bruises, including a black eye. Apply only to unbroken skin.

Baking soda (Sodium bicarbonate). Mix with water to form a paste and apply to insect bites and stings. It can also be applied to poison ivy. Used to make a rehydration drink.

Bandanna. Can be used to tie a splint or prevent chafing and blisters. Moisten and tie around head during the day to keep cool. Tuck into the back of your hat to shade the neck and protect it from sunburn. Can be moistened and used to protect the nose and mouth when traversing a fire area.

Bee sting kit. An absolute necessity if you or anyone in your household are allergic to beestings. Contains a spring-loaded syringe full of epinephrine or benadryl that prevents shock and reduces swelling.

Bromelain. An enzyme that occurs naturally in pineapple. Used to relieve swelling due to sports injuries, dental work, and surgery. You can take a 500-mg capsule 3 times a day. Must be taken 1 hour before meals or at least 3 hours after meals, or it acts as a digestive enzyme and loses its anti-inflammatory properties.

Castor oil. Apply to bruises.

Charcoal. Pure carbon capsules or powder. Can be taken internally for food poisoning, diarrhea, or gas or mushroom, drug, or chemical poisoning. (Do not give internally for poisoning unless suggested by a poison control center.) Charcoal can adsorb 40 times its weight, thus preventing poisons from entering the bloodstream. Mix with enough water to make a paste and use as a poultice on spider bites and infected wounds. *Do not use charcoal briquettes, which contain petrochemicals.*

Clay (green). Mix with water to make a paste and use as a poultice on bruises. Be sure to buy cosmetic quality green clay from a health food store, not the variety found in art stores.

Electrolyte beverage packets from health store. Turn to page 47 for instructions to make your own mix.

Essential oils. These are for topical use only and should be diluted in a carrier oil before being applied to the skin. Exceptions are lavender and tea tree oil, which can be applied without dilution. Pregnant women should avoid using essential oils even topically as their effect on pregnancy has not been tested yet.

> **Birch** *(Betula lenta)*. Relieves pain.
>
> **Calamus** *(Acorus calamus)*. For coma, memory, and head injury.
>
> **Citronella** *(Citronells nardus)*. Lemony smell repels insects.
>
> **Clove** *(Sygium aromaticum)*. Kills toothache. Contains eugenol, a natural anesthetic and antiseptic.
>
> **Eucalyptus** *(Eucalyptus globulus)*. Used in inhalations to loosen mucus and improve respiratory congestion. Antibacterial, antiviral, and decongestant.

Geranium *(Pelargonium graveolens)*. Reduces inflammation and prevents wound infection.

Ginger *(Zingiber officinale)*. Warming and anti-inflammatory.

Lavender *(Lavandula officinalis)*. For burns, headaches. Calms the nervous system when inhaled. Antiseptic and anti-inflammatory. Apply topically to wounds, burns, bruises, insect bites, and blisters. Reduces risk of infection and stimulates skin regeneration. Comforting to smell during the life transitions of birth and death.

Peppermint *(Mentha piperita)*. Cooling, antiseptic, aids digestive disorders; the aroma calms nausea. Can be used topically on burns and insect bites.

Rosemary *(Rosmarinus officinalis)*. For brain and memory impairment. Improves circulation and eases muscular pain. Antiseptic, aromatic.

Tea tree *(Melaleuca alternifolia)*. Apply topically to cuts, rashes, burns, bites, stings, fungal infection, sprains, and acne. Also works as an insect repellent. Two drops in a glass of water can be used as a gargle for sore throat. Antifungal, antiviral. One of the best nonirritating antiseptic essential oils.

Eye wash cup. For rinsing the eyes.

Herbal salve. For cuts and wounds. Look for a salve that has wound-healing herbs like calendula and comfrey along with infection-fighting ones such as myrrh, goldenseal, or echinacea. Or make the salve on page 131.

Herbs. When "herb" is listed as the plant part used, it means the entire above ground portion — leaf, flower, and stem. A * before the herb indicates the most important herbs to have in your first-aid kit because of multiple uses or profound emergency care use.

Agrimony leaf, flower, root *(Agrimonia eupatoria)*. Analgesic, anti-inflammatory, antispasmodic, antiviral, and lowers fever.

***Aloe vera** juice *(Aloe vera, A. ferox)*. Soothes inflammation, prevents fungus, heals wounds. Excellent for all burns, especially sunburn. Avoid internal use during pregnancy.

Angelica root *(Angelica archangelica, A. atropurpurea, A. officinalis)*. Stimulates uterine contractions and facilitates placenta delivery following the birth of a baby. Avoid internal use during pregnancy.

Blackberry leaf or root *(Rubus villosus)*. Astringent tea to stop diarrhea.

Black cohosh root, rhizome *(Cimicifuga racemosa)*. For seizures. Antispasmodic and muscle relaxant. Avoid during pregnancy.

Black haw bark *(Viburnum prunifolium)*. Astringent, antispasmodic.

Burdock root *(Arctium lappa)*. Antifungal and anti-inflammatory.

*****Calendula** flowers *(Calendula officinalis)*. Anti-inflammatory, antiseptic, and wound healing. Increases peripheral circulation.

Catnip leaf *(Nepeta cataria)*. Calms hysteria, pain, and seizures. Sedative.

*****Cayenne** pepper *(Capsicum frutescens)*. To stop bleeding internally and topically. It does sting to apply to bleeding wounds but is very effective. Take internally for frostbite and hypothermia. Blocks pain transmission and stimulates endorphin production. Antiseptic, hemostatic, and styptic. Both powder and tincture are effective.

*****Chamomile** flowers *(Matricaria recutita)*. Helps to calm and relieves stomach pains. Analgesic, antifungal, anti-inflammatory, antiseptic, antispasmodic, and sedative.

Cleavers herb *(Galium aparine)*. Blood and lymph cleansing. Bath herb for insect bites.

*****Comfrey** leaves *(Symphytum officinale)*. Poultice for bruises. Nowadays comfrey is generally used only topically rather than internally as there has been some concern about the pyrrolizidine alkaloids it contains. Avoid during pregnancy.

*****Echinacea** root, leaves, flowers, seed *(Echinacea purpurea, E. angustifolia)*. Used internally and topically for infection. Stimulates the immune system by increasing white blood cell production. For threatened colds, puncture wounds, and venomous bites. Antifungal, anti-inflammatory, antiseptic, antiviral, and wound healing.

*****Ephedra** stems *(Ephedra sinica)*. Bronchial dilator and circulatory stimulant. Effective in small doses in an emergency situation, but not to be used regularly or in dosages higher than recommended for those suffering from angina, diabetes, glaucoma, heart disease, high blood pressure, enlarged prostate gland, or overactive thyroid gland. Avoid during pregnancy.

*****Garlic** *(Allium sativum)*. Antifungal, antiparasitic, antiseptic, and immune stimulant.

*****Ginger** root *(Zingiber officinale)*. For motion sickness, morning sickness, stomachaches. Warming and inhibits prostaglandins. Improves circulation to all parts of the body. Anti-emetic and anti-inflammatory.

*****Goldenseal** root *(Hydrastis canadensis)*. Apply to wounds and bites to deter or treat infection. Also used internally. Effective against staph, strep, *E. coli*, salmonella, giardia, and candidia. Contricts blood vessels. Antiseptic and hemostatic. Please buy only goldenseal that has been cultivated as it is becoming endangered in the wild. Avoid during pregnancy.

Grindelia flower, bud (*Grindelia* spp.). Topically for poison ivy, oak, and sumac; also insect bites. Demulcent. Also known as Gumweed.

Jewelweed herb *(Impatiens aurens, I. pallida)*. Calms poison ivy itch. For topical use only.

Kelp *(Fucus vesiculosis)*. Helps prevent radiation from being absorbed by the body. Antioxidant and nutritive. Avoid long-term use in cases of hyperthyroidism.

Lemon balm herb *(Melissa officinalis)*. Antidepressant, antiviral, and sedative.

Marshmallow root *(Althaea officinalis)*. Demulcent, nutritive, and wound healing.

Milk thistle seed *(Silybum marianum)*. Helps protect the liver from damage from chemical exposure.

Nettles herb*(Urtica dioica, U. urens)*. Rich in trace minerals that help in bone and skin repair. Nutritive.

Oatstraw herb *(Avena sativa)*. Nerve tonic. Helps build healthy bones and skin. Nutritive.

****Peppermint** leaf *(Mentha piperita)*. Cooling herb, benefits digestion, can be used in the bath to calm itching. Compress for fevers, heatstroke.

****Plantain** leaves *(Plantago major, P. lanceolata)*. Promotes blood coagulation and wound healing. For wounds, bleeding, poison ivy, and snakebites. Anti-inflammatory, antiseptic, and hemostatic.

Raspberry leaf *(Rubus* spp.). Hemostatic, nutritive, uterine tonic. Facilitates birth and placental delivery.

Red clover blossoms *(Trifolium pratense)*. Promotes wound healing and aids the body's natural systems of detoxification.

Red root *(Ceanothus americanus)*. Lymph and blood cleansing.

Reishi mushrooms *(Ganoderma lucidum)*. Aid in the prevention of and recovery from illness. Calms the mind and spirit. Antiseptic, immune stimulant.

Rosemary herb *(Rosmarinus officinalis)*. Antiseptic. Calms anxiety, improves headaches and digestion. Avoid therapeutic doses during pregnancy.

Sage herb *(Salvia officinalis)*. Antifungal and antiseptic. Avoid during pregnancy.

St.-John's-wort herb *(Hypericum perforatum).* Helps heal damaged nerves. May cause photosensitivity in some individuals.

*****Shepherd's purse** leaf *(Capsella bursa-pastoris).* Constricts blood vessels. Avoid during pregnancy.

Skullcap herb *(Scutellaria lateriflora).* Encourages endorphin production and sedates the brain and spinal column. Antispasmodic, nervine, and sedative.

Turmeric root *(Curcuma longa).* Anti-inflammatory and circulatory stimulant. Avoid during pregnancy.

*****Valerian** root *(Valeriana officinalis).* For pain, anxiety, and insomnia. Antispasmodic, muscle relaxant, and sedative.

White oak bark *(Quercus alba).* Anti-inflammatory, antiseptic, and astringent. Bath herb for insect bites.

*****Yarrow** herb *(Achillea millefolium).* Stops bleeding and lowers fever. Avoid during pregnancy.

Yellow dock root *(Rumex crispus).* Improves the function of the kidneys, liver, lymph, and intestines.

Homeopathic remedies. Homeopathic remedies are usually taken by placing 4 pellets under the tongue every 4 hours for the first few days following an injury. And although some of their ingredients in large amounts could be toxic, they are so diluted that what you are getting is the "energy" of the remedy that can help stimulate the body's own healing process. In the following list, the source of the remedy is in parentheses. Homeopathic medicines use minute doses; be aware that some of the substances used could be toxic in larger amounts. Stick with the homeopathic dose.

Acetic acid (glacial acetic acid). For cat bites.

**Aconitum* *(Aconitum napellus,* Monkshood). Helps relieve bleeding. It can be used to help shock and the trauma that results from sudden injury. Helps patients who are anxious and fearful when they are experiencing nausea and vomiting.

Antimonium tartaricum (tartrate of antimony and potash). Administered after a near-drowning episode to a victim who's too weak to cough.

**Apis* *(Apis mellifica,* honeybee). Beestings, insect bites. For bites or stings that result in hot, puffy conditions and sensitivity to touch, that are improved by cold applications and worsened by heat. *Apis* is also suggested for rashes, frostbite, and the initial stages of boils.

Arnica (*Arnica montana* flower). For shock, trauma (physical and emotional), pain, bruises, black eyes, swelling, muscle injury, before and after surgery, dentistry, and labor. Usually the first remedy given after a traumatic event. Arnica is also used before and after surgery to minimize swelling and speed healing. Aids in reabsorption of fibrin, a blood protein that forms as a result of internal injuries, thereby reducing swelling and bruising. Use *Arnica* salve or liniment for sore muscles, bruises, sprains, black eye, torn ligaments. Don't use arnica oil topically on broken skin as it can cause irritation and bleeding.

Arsenicum (Arsenicum album, arsenic trioxide). Can help poisoning when there is intense vomiting along with restlessness and anxiety. Helps food poisoning. Relieves burning abdominal pain, diarrhea, and vomiting. Also helps rashes that come on suddenly.

Belladonna (deadly nightshade). Use for early stages of food poisoning. Patient may be flushed and feverish. Symptoms come on suddenly.

Bellis (*Bellis perennis,* daisy). For bruises, soreness, and to ease pain and speed recovery after an injury.

Byronia (Wild hops). For broken bones, injuries to bones, ribs, and discs. Good for injuries when the slightest movement hurts and continued motion does not help.

Cantharis (Spanish fly). For painful burns and scalds, before blisters form.

Carbo vegetabilis (vegetable charcoal). For newborn baby with bluish skin who has not yet established strong breathing; also for heat stroke in cases of extreme exhaustion.

Chamomilla (German chamomile). Calming, for toothache pain.

Coffea (Coffea cruda, unroasted coffee). Calms overexcitement; for intense, stinging toothache.

Euphrasia (eyebright). Alleviates itching, irritation, and inflammation in the eyes.

Ferrum phosphoricum (phosphate of iron). To stop a nosebleed.

Hepar sulph (hepar sulfuris calcareum, or calcium sulfide). For splinters, tooth infection.

Hypericum (St.-John's-wort). For wounds, nerve injury to areas with lots of nerves such as fingers, toes, and spine. Can help prevent the need for stitches. For crushing injuries and sharp shooting pain. For old injuries with nerves that still hurt. Use after dental work.

Ipecac (Ipecacuanha, ipecac root). Extreme, persistent nausea. For arterial bleeding. Cold and anxious. Little thirst.

Lachesis (bushmaster snake). For dog bites.

*Ledum (marsh tea). For puncture wounds, insect (mosquito) and animal bites, and black eyes. Sprains, fractures, stiff joints, lingering bruises, and cold and numb feelings.

Magnesia phosphorica (phosphate of magnesia). For toothache with intense, piercing pain shooting along the nerve; also for heat exhaustion.

*Nux vomica (poison nut). For nausea that is relieved from moving bowels, causes chilliness after vomiting, or is caused by overindulgence.

Phosphorus (Phosphorus). For jet lag, when feeling dizzy, sluggish, and absentminded.

*Rhus tox (*Rhus toxicodendron,* poison ivy). For sprains, strains, and stiffness. For injuries that are worse upon initial movement, but then feel better after continued movement. For dislocated joints, ligaments, and muscle pain. For joints that are hot, swollen, and painful. Also helps to relieve poison ivy, rashes.

*Ruta graveolens (rue). For sprains, torn tendons, and injuries to bone coverings (the periosteum). Use for bone pain and bruises; blows to elbow, knee, and shin. Use after *Arnica,* 24 hours later if help is still needed. Use when cold air makes injury feel worse.

Spongia tosta (roasted sponge). For loud wheezing during an asthma attack.

Staphysagria (Stavesacre). For swelling related to insect bites and stings. Also for toothache due to decay.

Sulphur (sublimated sulphur). For poison ivy with a burning itch.

*Symphytum (comfrey). For fractures and injuries to cheekbone and eye area. Speeds up healing for bone injuries.

*Urtica urens (stinging nettle). For burns.

*Veratrum (*Veratrum album,* white hellebore). For bleeding, on the verge of shock.

Vespa (wasp). For wasp stings.

Honey. An antiseptic that can be applied topically to cuts and burns. Avoid giving internally to children under two years of age.

Ipecac syrup *(Cephaelis ipecacuanha).* For use when directed by a poison control center to induce vomiting. Ipecac is a South American shrub that contains emetine, an alkaloid that induces vomiting. Ipecac stimulates gastric secretions, which activates the brain's vomiting reflex.

Insect Repellent. Use one made with essential plant oils (see page 38). Applied to skin to deter a wide range of bugs.

Latex gloves. To protect yourself against blood-borne pathogens when treating wounds.

Liquid soap. To clean wounds. Consider having an antiseptic soap that contains tea tree or lavender essential oils.

Pantothenic acid (vitamin B_5). Helps reduce swelling from beestings and allergic reactions.

Papain. An enzyme that occurs naturally in unripe papaya. Aids in protein digestion and when applied topically helps break down the large protein molecules in bee venom.

Povidone iodine. The new replacement for that old standby, hydrogen peroxide. Used topically to disinfect wounds.

Rescue Remedy. For shock, panic, fear, trauma. Also sometimes marketed under other names such as Five Flower Remedy. (See page 19 for more information.)

Sea salt. Used to make rehydration drink (see recipe on page 47). Add one pound (454 g) to bath for insect bites. Can be used as a mouth rinse for toothache.

St.-John's-wort oil *(Hypericum perforatum)*. For burn application and nerve injury.

Tape. For holding bandages together.

Tweezers. For removing splinters, thorns, and other foreign objects.

Ume concentrate or umeboshi plum paste *(Prunus mume)*. For food poisoning, diarrhea, constipation, acid indigestion, motion sickness, headache, hangover, fatigue, dysentery, typhoid, and parasite prevention. "Don't leave home without it." Made from a fermented plum.

Vinegar. Can be applied to sunburn, bee sting, spider bites, and jellyfish sting and mixed with baking soda to make a paste for bee stings. Apple cider vinegar is considered the most therapeutic.

Vitamin C. Helps the body better resist infection. Can help reduce allergic reactions, including those to foods, animals, insect bites, and stings.

Vitamin E. A natural antioxidant that can aid tissue repair. When applied topically to burns and wounds can help prevent scar formation. It is also wise to take it internally during periods of healing.

TRAVELING FIRST-AID KIT

You can't lug your entire herbal first-aid kit around. So here's a list of multiuse essentials to keep in your handbag or briefcase.

Echinacea tincture	Homeopathic *Arnica*
Rescue Remedy	Lavender essential oil
Herbal salve	Tea tree essential oil
Adhesive dressings	Ume concentrate

SURVIVAL KIT FOR THE CAR

A snowstorm strikes unexpectedly. A flash flood washes away the road. Ten people are injured in a multi-car crash on the expressway. These are things that happen every day in every part of the world. To be prepared to handle them, here's what you should keep in your car:

Ax. To chop wood. Can be of aid in constructing a makeshift shelter.
Blanket. In case you need to bivouac in the cold. Also useful in treatment of shock.
Candles.
Carborundum. This is a small stone used to keep knives and tools sharp.
Clothes. Sweaters, socks, shoes, hat, and gloves.
Compass.
Cooking pot.
Fire extinguisher.
First-aid book. Preferably a second copy of this one.
Fishhook and line.
Flares.
Flashlight with extra batteries.
Flint. Can be used after you run out of matches to start a fire. Get a processed flint with a saw striker.
Food. Dried food is easiest to store, but it needs water to be reconstituted.
Glasses. If you wear them, having an extra pair could be lifesaving.
Knife.
Magnifying glass. Could be used to start a fire or to locate an embedded splinter or stinger.

Map.

Matches, waterproof. Store in waterproof containers and prevent them from rolling and rattling together. In rare instances, that kind of contact could cause them to ignite.

Paper and pencil. So you can leave messages or information of your whereabouts.

Pepper spray. Can be used to defend oneself from attackers — people as well as animals.

Plastic bag. Large bags can be used as a solar still, water container, and emergency rain poncho. Can also keep your supplies dry. Smaller zip-type bags can be used to hold water or soak wounds.

Quarters and dimes. To make phone calls.

Radio (battery-operated). To listen for instructions and warnings about natural or man-made disasters. Be sure to have a supply of extra batteries.

Rope. For towing, rescue, and tying things together.

Saw. Flexible varieties are available that don't take up much room. Can be used for fire and shelter building.

Sewing kit. To repair clothes, sleeping gear, and tents. Have at least some large-eye needles that can be threaded with coarse thread as well as the regular varieties of needles and thread.

Shovel. For digging a shelter, fire pit, digging out of snow, collecting edible roots.

Sleeping bag.

Snakebite kit. Especially if traveling in areas where snakes are known to reside. Keep a kit in your pocket when out hiking.

Water container. Collapsible is fine. To fetch or store water. If empty and closed, can be used as flotation device.

Water purification tablets or water filter.

Whistle. To maintain contact with your party, to conserve your voice when needing to signal for help.

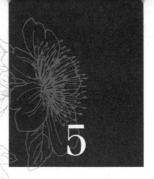

HOW TO MAKE AND USE HERBAL MEDICINES

Herbs are God's gift to the earth and its inhabitants. When they are made into teas, tinctures, salves, poultices, and compresses, they frequently allow us to heal ourselves of everyday bangs, bruises, and bumps. Here's how they are made and used.

HERBAL TEAS

An herbal tea made from leaves or flowers is called an *infusion*. To make an infusion, bring 1 cup (230 ml) of pure water to a boil in a nonaluminum pot and remove from heat. Add 1 heaping teaspoon (5 ml) of dried herb or 2 teaspoons (10 ml) fresh. Cover. Let sit for at least 10 minutes. Strain. Use immediately, or store in the refrigerator and use within 4 days.

An herbal tea made from roots and barks is called a *decoction*. One caveat: If a root is particularly high in volatile oils (such as ginger or valerian) it is best infused rather than decocted. To make a decoction, simmer 1 heaping teaspoon (5 ml) of dried herb or 2 teaspoons (10 ml) fresh in 1 cup (230 ml) water while covered for 20 minutes. Strain. Use immediately, or store in the refrigerator and use within 4 days.

Once strained from the liquid, spent herbs can be returned to the earth by mixing them in with your compost or garden soil.

The Secrets of a Professional Herbalist

Ever wonder why a professional herbalist's preparations are so good? Here are a few rules of thumb that professionals use when buying, making, and storing herbs:

- Buy quality herbs from reputable suppliers.
- Buy herbs in bulk and store in glass jars away from light and heat.
- When a recipe calls for parts, measure the ingredient by weight, not volume.
- Make small batches the first time around.
- Prepare herbs in containers and with utensils made of glass, stainless steel, or ceramic. Other materials, such as plastic, copper, or aluminum can contaminate the products.
- Label every herbal preparation with the ingredients, how it should be used, and the date it was made. Generally speaking, capsules will last about two years, and tinctures about five years.

HERBAL TINCTURES

Tinctures are easy to store and use. They have traditionally been made on the new moon so that the energy of the moon can draw out the properties of the herbs.

Prepare the herbs by chopping or grinding them. You may tincture several herbs together if you are creating a formula. Then put the herb in a glass jar and cover with vodka. The alcohol you use must be at least 50 proof to have good preservative qualities.

Store the tincture away from light and shake it once a day for a month. Then strain, first with a strainer and then through a clean, undyed cloth, squeezing tightly. Bottle in dark glass bottles. Add spent herbs to the compost. Label and date the tincture — they'll keep for at least five years. Store away from heat and light. Take tinctures by putting 1 dropperful in a bit of warm water and drinking.

Tinctures may also be made using vegetable glycerin rather than alcohol. This is best when making tinctures for those that are alcohol intolerant as well as for children and pregnant and nursing mothers. Glycerin is more effective than water but less effective than alcohol. It is naturally sweet and pleasant tasting, and is slightly antiseptic, demulcent, and healing when diluted. Tinctures made with glycerin, called glycerites, are usually prepared in the same manner as alcohol-based tinctures but using 1 part water to 2 parts glycerin. Glycerites have a shorter shelf life than tinctures prepared with alcohol, about one to three years.

A HEALING POULTICE

A poultice is the herb applied directly to the skin. Crush a fresh or dried herb and mix with hot water, apple cider vinegar, or olive or castor oil, depending on what your needs are and what is available. The liquid helps to hold the herbs together and in place.

Apply the poultice to the area of the body needing attention, such as a wound. Possible poultices include:
- Chopped cabbage to draw out pus and toxins
- Chopped carrot for bruises, chapped skin
- Comfrey for swellings, sores, and wounds
- Oatmeal for inflammation and insect bites

If using dried instead of fresh herbs, you can add cornmeal or freshly ground flaxseed to thicken the paste.

Poultices may be reapplied several times a day or in succession during one sitting. A cloth or comfrey or plantain leaves can be applied to help hold the poultice in place. Mustard will cause the skin to blister, so should never be applied directly to the skin, but placed *on* a cloth.

COMPRESSES

Compresses are made by soaking a clean towel in hot or cold herbal tea. The cloth is then wrung out and applied to the area needing treatment. Covering the wet cloth with a dry towel will help the cloth to stay hot or cold. When the compress temperature changes (the hot cools down, for example), resoak the cloth in the tea and reapply. This can be repeated.

Cold often is best for hot, inflamed conditions such as swellings or a headache. Hot compresses are good for backache, arthritic pain, and sore throats. The best indicator is to ask the person needing treatment if they think cold or hot will give the best relief.

An Herbal Healing Salve

There are many different herbs that can be used in a salve. Below is an example of a formula that will help to speed wound healing and prevent infection. Apply salves several times a day as needed. It is best to use dried herbs, as moisture from fresh plants can cause the salve to spoil more quickly.

½ ounce (14 g) comfrey root, cut and sifted
¼ ounce (7 g) calendula blossoms
¼ ounce (7 g) plantain leaves
¼ ounce (7 g) myrrh resin
¼ ounce (7 g) echinacea, goldenseal (not wild-crafted), usnea, or propolis, finely cut
½ cup (115 ml) olive oil
¼ ounce (7 g) grated beeswax
4 drops gum benzoin tincture (available from drugstores)
Up to 40 drops essential oil (lavender, rosemary, or peppermint)
2 400-IU vitamin E capsules

1. Put herbs and olive oil into a slow cooker, set heat to low, and cook overnight. The next day, turn off the heat and allow the mixture to cool.

2. Strain the herbs out of the oil through a strainer and then through a clean, natural fiber cloth, squeezing it tightly. Return the oil to the cooker and set heat to high. Add the grated beeswax. When it has melted, mix well and remove from heat. Stir in the benzoin, essential oil, and the liquid contents of the vitamin E capsules.

3. Test 1 teaspoon (5 ml) of the product by putting it in a container and letting it cool and harden to see what the final consistency will be. If it is too soft to work as a salve, you may need to add a bit more beeswax. If it is too hard, add a bit more oil.

4. Pour your salve into clean, dry glass or ceramic containers. Be sure to date and label your containers.

INDEX

Page references in *italics* indicate illustrations.

Abdominal injuries, 20–21.
  See also Stomach pain
Abrasions and lacerations,
  21–24, *22*
Acetic acid, for cat bites, 26, 122
Acidophilus
  for burns, 42
  for diaper rash, 46
  for diarrhea, 47
  for food poisoning, 57
Aconitum, 122
  for bleeding, severe, 24
  for drowning, shock from,
    49
Acupressure
  for diarrhea, 48
  for seizures or convulsions, 76
  for toothache, 90
  for vomiting, 92
Agaricus, for frostbite numb-
    ness, 60
Agrimony, 119
  for stomach pain, 87
Alcohol poisoning, 24. *See also*
  CPR; Drug/alcohol over-
  dose
Allergic reaction, 25. *See also*
  Hives; Stings
Aloe vera, 119
  for burns, 40
  for frostbite, 60
  for hives, 66
  for jellyfish stings, 68
  for poison ivy, oak, sumac, 74
  for radiation, 113
  for sunburn, 89
Anacardium 3x, for poison ivy,
  oak, sumac, 74
Angostura bitters, for hangover, 51
Angelica, 119
Animal bites and scratches,
  25–26
Ankle injury. *See* Sprains and
  strains
Antimonium tartaricum, for
  drowning, 49, 122

Apis, 122
  for frostbite, 59
  for hot, stingy wounds, 26
  for stings, insect, 85
Apple cider vinegar, 125
  for ant bites, 36
  for bruises, 35
  for bug bites, 36, 37
  for diaper rash, 45
  for nosebleed, 70
  for poison ivy, oak, sumac,
    73, 74
  for spider bites, 81
  for sprains and strains, 82
  for stingray stings, 84
  for sunburn, 88
  for vomiting, 92
Apples
  for chemical contamination,
    43
  for diarrhea, 47
  for food poisoning, 57
  for radiation, 113
Arnica, 117, 123
  for black eye, 31
  for bruises, 35
  for childbirth, 97
  for frostbite, shock, 60
  for shock, 78
  for snakebite, 80
  for sprains and strains, 82
Arsenicum, 123
  for asthma attack, mild, 28
  for burned skin, 41
  for diarrhea, 48
  for drowning, anxiety from,
    49
Artemesia, for poison ivy, oak,
  sumac, 74
Asthma, 27–28
Avalanche survival, 93–94
Avocados, for heat stroke, 64
Back and neck injuries, 8, 18,
  29
Baking soda, 117
  for allergic reaction, 25
  for bug bites, 36, 37
  for eyes, burns, 53

  for hives, 65
  for poison ivy, oak, sumac, 74
  for radiation, 113
  for stingray stings, 84
  for stings, insect, 85
  for sunburn, 88
Bananas
  for bruises, 35
  for heat stroke, 64
Bananas, Rice, Applesauce,
  Tea/Toast (BRAT), for
  diarrhea, 47
Bandaging limbs, 16
B-complex
  for hangover, 51
  for seizures or convulsions,
    76
Bear, encounter with a, 94–95
Bee propolis, for abrasions and
  lacerations, 23
Bee stings, 29–30, 118. *See also*
  Stings
Belladonna, 123
  for toothache, 90
Bellis, 123
  for bruises with swelling, 35
Beta carotene
  for asthma, 28
  for burns, 42
Birch essential oil, 118
  for sprains and strains, 82
Birth, 96–101
Blackberry, for diarrhea, 47, 119
Black cohosh, for seizures, 76,
  119
Black eye, 30–31
Black haw, 119
  for threatened miscarriage,
    100
Black tea
  for drug/alcohol overdose, 50
  for poisoning, 72
  for sunburn, 88
Black walnut, for electric
  shock, 52
Bleeding, 31–33, *32. See also*
  Abrasions and lacerations;
  Nosebleed

Blisters, 33
Blue-green algae, for burns, 42
Bones, broken. *See* Fractures;
    Splints and slings
BRAT (Bananas, Rice,
    Applesauce, Tea/Toast),
    for diarrhea, 47
Breathing difficulties, 3,
    33–34. *See also* Asthma;
    CPR; Heimlich Maneuver
Bromelain, 118
    for frostbite, 60
    for sprains and strains, 83
    for stings, insect, 86
Bruises, 34–36
Bug bites, 36–38. *See also*
    Spider bites; Stings
Bull charge survival, 95
Burdock
    for chemical contamina-
        tion, 44
    for poison ivy, oak, sumac,
        73, 74
    for sprains and strains, 82
Burdock *(Arctium lappa),* 119
Burns, 39–42. *See also* Eyes,
    heat and chemical burns;
    Sunburn
Buttermilk, for poison ivy,
    oak, sumac, 74
Byronia, 123
    for heat stroke, 64
    for sprains and strains, 83
Cabbage
    for bruises, 35
    for sprains and strains, 82
Calamus essential oil, 118
    for head injury, mental
        functions, 61
Calcium
    for fractures, 58
    for seizures or convulsions,
        76
    for sprains and strains, 83
Calendula, 119
    for abrasions and lacera-
        tions, 23
    for animal bites and
        scratches, 26
    for diaper rash, 45
    for hives, 66
    for poison ivy, oak, sumac,
        73
    for tick bites, 37

Cantaloupe, for heat stroke, 64
Cantharis, 123
    for sunburn, 89
    for third-degree burns, 40
Car accident survival, 95–96,
    120–21
Carbo vegetabilis, 123
    for heat stroke, 64
Cardiopulmonary
    Resuscitation (CPR),
    3–10, *5–8,*
Carob powder, for diarrhea,
    47
Carrots
    for burns, 40
    for chemical contamina-
        tion, 43
    for diarrhea, 47
    for radiation, 113
Castor oil, 118
    for stomach pain, 87
Catnip, 120
    for seizures or convulsions,
        76
Cayenne pepper, 120
    for abrasions and lacera-
        tions, 23
    after childbirth, 99–100
    for cold (severe), 101
    for heart attack, 63
    for nosebleed, 70
    for sprains and strains, 82
Cedarwood essential oil, for
    bug bites, 38
Chamomile, 120
    for hives, 66
    for stomach pain, 87
    for sunburn, 89
Chamomilla, 123
    for diarrhea, 48
    for toothache, 90
Chaparral, for abrasions and
    lacerations, 23
Charcoal, 118
    for diarrhea, 47
    for drug/alcohol overdose,
        50
    for food poisoning, 56
    for poisoning, 71, 72
Chemical contamination,
    43–44. *See also* Eyes, heat
    and chemical burns
Childbirth, 96–101
Chile pepper, for frostbite, 59

Ching Wan Hung, for burns, 41
Chlorella
    for burns, 42
    for seizures or convulsions,
        76
Chlorophyll
    for asthma, 28
    for radiation, 113
Choking, 11, *11,* 34, 44–45.
    See also Heimlich
    Maneuver
Cider, spiced, for hypother-
    mia, 67
Cinnamon bark, for diarrhea,
    47
Citronella essential oil, for
    bug repellent, 38, 118
Clay. *See* Green clay
Cleavers, 120
    for bug bites, 37
Clorox, for water purification,
    114
Clove essential oil, for
    toothache, 90, 118
Coenzyme Q10, for frostbite,
    60
Coffea, 123
    for toothache, 90
Coffee, for drug/alcohol over-
    dose, 50
Cold compress
    for asthma attack, 27
    for black eye, 30
    for bruises, 34
    for burns, 40, 42
    for heat stroke, 63, 64
    for nosebleed, 69
    for snakebite, 79
    for sprains and strains, 82
Cold (severe) survival, 101–2.
    See also Fire making;
    Frostbite; Hypothermia
Comfrey, 120
    for bruises, 35
    for burns, 40, 42
    for sprains and strains, 82
Compresses, 130
Convulsions or seizures,
    75–77. *See also* CPR
Cornstarch
    for bug bites, 37
    for hives, 66
    for poison ivy, oak, sumac,
        74

CPR (Cardiopulmonary Resuscitation), 3–10, *5–8,* 9
Crab, for burns, 42
Cranesbill, for abrasions and lacerations, 23
Cucumber
    for ant bites, 36
    for burns, 41
    for heat stroke, 64
    for sunburn, 89
Cuts. *See* Abrasions and lacerations
Dandelion
    for chemical contamination, 44
    for food, 109
    for hives, 66
    for poison ivy, oak, sumac, 74
Decoctions, 128
Dehydration, 116. *See also* Electrolyte rehydration drink
DHA, for stroke, 88
Diaper rash, 45–46
Diarrhea, 46–48
Drowning, 49. *See also* CPR; Recovery position
Drug/alcohol overdose, 50–51. *See also* Alcohol poisoning; CPR; Recovery position
Ear injury, 51
Earthquake survival, 102
Echinacea, 120
    for abrasions and lacerations, 23, 24
    for animal bites and scratches, 26
    for blisters, 33
    for burns, 42
    for caterpillar bites, 36
    for ear injury, 51
    for food poisoning, 57
    for jellyfish stings, 68
    for scorpion stings, 75
    for snakebite, 80
    for stingray stings, 84
    for stings, insect, 85
    for stomach pain, 87
    for tick bites, 37
    for ticks, 36
Electric shock, 52. *See also* CPR
Electrolyte rehydration drink, 119

for burns, 40
for diarrhea, 46, 47
for fever, 55
for heat stroke, 64
for shock, 78
Ephedra, 120
    for allergic reaction, 25
    for hives, 65
Epinephrine
    for bee stings, 30
    for stings, insect, 84, 86
Essential fatty acids, for fractures, 58
Eucalyptus essential oil, 118
    for bug bites, 38
    for frostbite, 60
Euphrasia, 123
    for black eye, 31
    for eyes, burns, 53
Eyes, heat and chemical burns, 39, 53
Fainting, 53–54. *See also* CPR; Recovery position; Unconsciousness
Fenugreek, for asthma, 28
Ferrum phosphoricum, for nosebleed, 70, 123
Fever, 55
Fire making, 104–5
Fire survival, 103–5. *See also* Burns
First-aid kits, 117–27
First-degree burns, 39, 40–42
Flood survival, 105–6. *See also* Water shortage survival
Food foraging, 109–10
Food poisoning, 56–57. *See also* Stomach pain
Fractures, 57–58. *See also* Splints and slings
Frostbite, 58–60. *See also* Cold (severe) survival; Fire making; Hypothermia
Garlic, 120
    for asthma, 28
    for bug bites, 38
    for drowning, lung infections, 49
    for food poisoning, 57
    for hypothermia, 67
    for scorpion stings, 75
    for snakebite, 80
    for spider bites, 81
    for toothache, 89

Gelsenium, for heat stroke, 64
Geranium essential oil, 118
    for bug bites, 38
    for frostbite, 60
Ginger, 120
    for asthma, lung circulation, 27
    for bruises, 35
    for diarrhea, 47
    for fever, 55
    for food poisoning, 56
    for frostbite, 59
    for hypothermia, 67
    for sprains and strains, 82
    for stomach pain, 87
    for toothache, 90
    for vomiting, 92
Ginger ale, for vomiting, 92
Ginger essential oil, 119
    for frostbite, 60
Ginkgo
    for drowning, oxygen utilization, 49
    for stroke, 88
Glonoine, for heat stroke, 64
Glycerites, 130
Goldenseal, 120
    for abrasions and lacerations, 23
    for poison ivy, oak, sumac, 73
Gotu kola
    for abrasions and lacerations, 24
    for stroke, 88
Green clay, 118
    for ant bites, 36
    for bruises, 35
    for chemical contamination, 43
    for diarrhea, 47
    for food poisoning, 56
    for poison ivy, oak, sumac, 73
    for sprains and strains, 82
    for stings, insect, 85
Green tea, for sunburn, 88
Grindelia, for poison ivy, oak, sumac, 73, 121
Head injury, 60–61. *See also* Bleeding; Unconsciousness
Heart attack, 4, 62–63. *See also* CPR; Recovery position
Heat stroke, 63–65

Heimlich Maneuver, 11–16, 12–16
Hepar sulph, 123
  for toothache, 90
Herbal
  insect repellent, 38
  medicines, 128–31
  salve, 23, 122, 131
  teas, 128
  tinctures, 129–30
Hibiscus, for heat stroke, 64
Hives, 65–66. *See also* Allergic reaction
Homeopathic dosages, 19
Honey, 124
  for burns, 41, 42
  for hangover, 51
Hypericum, 123
  for black eye, 31
  for bruises to sensitive areas, 35
  for burns and nerve damage, 41
  for frostbite, nerve damage, 60
  for wounds with severe pain, 24
Hypothermia, 66–67. *See also* Cold (severe) survival; Fire making; Frostbite

Ice rescue, 106. *See also* Drowning; Hypothermia
Immobilization, applying splints and slings, 16–17, 17
Infants and children, CPR for, 8–10, 9
Insect bites. *See* Bug bites; Scorpion stings; Spider bites; Stings
Ipecac, 124
  for asthma, excess mucus, 28
Ipecac syrup, for poisoning, 71, 124
Jellyfish stings, 67–68
Jewelweed, 121
  for nettle rash, 68
  for poison ivy, oak, sumac, 73
Jing Wan Hong, for burns, 41
Kelp, for radiation, 113, 121
Lacerations and abrasions, 21–24, 22
Lachesis, 124
  for dog bites, 26

  for frostbite, feet, 60
Lavender essential oil, 119
  for abrasions and lacerations, 23
  for animal bites and scratches, 26
  for blisters, 33
  for bruises, 35
  for bug bites, 38
  for burns, 40
  for caterpillar bites, 36
  for fainting, 54
  for fever, 55
  for heat stroke, 64
  for jellyfish stings, 68
  for mosquito bites, 36
  for nosebleed, 69
  for scorpion stings, 75
  for shock, 78
  for spider bites, 81
  for stings, insect, 85
  for sunburn, 88
  for unconsciousness, 91
Lecithin, for seizures or convulsions, 76
Ledum, 124
  for bites, deep, 26
  for black eye, 31
  for bruises with tenderness, 35
  for fractures, 58
  for poison ivy, oak, sumac, 74
  for puncture wounds with swelling, 24
  for sprains and strains, 83
Lemon, for vomiting, 92
Lemon balm, 121
  for heat stroke, 64
Lemon juice, for mosquito bites, 36
Lightning survival, 106–7
Limbs, bandaging, 16
Lime, for scorpion stings, 75
Lipoic acid, for stroke, 88
Lobelia
  for asthma, lung spasms, 28
  for burns, 42
Lost in wilderness survival, 107–10. *See also* Fire making
Lyme disease, 37
Magnesia phosphorica, 124
  for heat stroke, 64
  for toothache, 90

Magnesium
  for fractures, 58
  for seizures or convulsions, 76
  for sprains and strains, 83
Marshmallow root, 121
  for burns, 42
  for throats, irritated, 45
Massage
  after childbirth, 100
  for seizures or convulsions, 76
  for vomiting, 92
Medicines, herbal, 128–31
Milk
  for poisoning, 71
  for stings, insect, 85
  for sunburn, 89
Milk of magnesia, for poisoning, 72
Milk thistle, for chemical contamination, 44, 121
Mint leaf, for nettle rash, 68
Miscarriage, 100
Miso soup
  for chemical contamination, 43
  for diarrhea, 47
  for food poisoning, 57
  for radiation, 113
Mountain lion, encounter with a, 110–11
Moving the injured, 18–19
Mud
  for ant bites, 36
  for mosquito bites, 36
  for stings, insect, 85
Mullein leaf, for nettle rash, 68
Mung bean soup, for burns, 42
Mustard, for toothache, 90
Myrrh, for poison ivy, oak, sumac, 73
Natrum sulphuricum, for head injury, 61
Neck injuries, 8, 18, 29
Nettle rash, 68
Nettles, 121
  after childbirth, 100
  for burns, 42
  for hives, 66
  for nosebleed, 70
  for poison ivy, oak, sumac, 74
Niacin, for frostbite, 60

Nosebleed, 69–70
Nux vomica, 124
　for diarrhea, 48
　for vomiting, 92
Oatmeal
　for diarrhea, 47
　for hives, 66
　for hypothermia, 67
　for poison ivy, oak, sumac, 74
Oatstraw, 121
　for fever, 55
　for heat stroke, 64
Onion
　for asthma, 28
　for bruises, 35
　for sprains and strains, 82
　for stings, insect, 85
Osha, for abrasions and lacer-
　ations, 23
Panothenic acid (vitamin B$_5$)
　125
Papain powder, for insect
　stings, 85, 125
Papaya, for stingray stings, 84
Parsley, for bruises, 35
Peppermint, 121
　for bug bites, 37
　for food poisoning, 56
　for stomach pain, 87
　for sunburn, 89
　for vomiting, 92
Peppermint essential oil, 119
　for bug bites, 36
　for fainting, 54
　for fever, 55
　for heat stroke, 64
　for shock, 78
　for sunburn, 88
　for unconsciousness, 91
Phosphorus, 124
　for diarrhea, 48
　for electric shock, 52
　for small wounds and heavy
　　bleeding, 24
Phytochemicals, for sprains
　and strains, 82
Pine resin, for toothache, 90
Plantain, 121
　for ant bites, 36
　for black eye, 31
　for bruises, 23
　for burns, 40
　for hives, 66
　for mosquito bites, 36

　for nettle rash, 68
　for poison ivy, oak, sumac, 73
　for sprains and strains, 82
　for stings, insect, 85
　for toothache, 90
Podophyllin, for diarrhea, 48
Poisoning, 70–72. *See also*
　Food poisoning
Poison ivy, oak, sumac, 72–74
Porcupine, encounter with a,
　111
Potassium, for sprains and
　strains, 83
Potatoes
　for black eye, 31
　for bruises, 35
　for burns, 40
　for heat stroke, 64
　for sprains and strains, 82
Poultices, 130
　for ant bites, 36
　for black eye, 31
　for bruises, 35
　for burns, 40
　for poison ivy, oak, sumac, 73
　for snakebite, 80
　for toothache, 90
Povidone iodine, 125
Pregnancy, and imminent
　childbirth, 96–101
Psyllium seed, for diarrhea, 47
Pulse, stopping of, 3. *See also*
　CPR
Quercetin, for insect stings, 86
Quicksand survival, 111
Rabies survival, 111–12
Radiation survival, 112–13
Raspberry, 121
　for diarrhea, 47
Recovery position, 18, *18*
Red clover, 121
　for burns, 42
　for chemical contamination,
　　44
　for hives, 66
　for poison ivy, oak, sumac, 74
Red root, 121
Rehydration drink. *See* Electro-
　lyte rehydration drink
Reishi mushroom, 121
　for stress, 44
Rescue Remedy, 125
　for abdominal injuries, 21
　for burns, shock from, 41

　for drowning, shock from, 49
　for fainting, 54
　for head injury, 61
　ingredients of, 19
　for seizures or convulsions,
　　76
　for shock, 78
Rhus tox, 124
　for bruises with swelling, 35
　for poison ivy, oak, sumac, 74
　for sprains and strains, 83
Rocky Mountain spotted
　fever, 37
Rosemary, 121
　for nettle rash, 68
Rosemary essential oil, 119
　for bug bites, 38
　for fainting, 54
　for head injury, mental
　　functions, 61
　for shock, 78
Ruta graveolens, 124
　for bruises to bones, 35
　for sprains and strains, 83
Sage, 121
　for nettle rash, 68
Salt, for toothache, 89
Salve, herbal, 23, 122, 131
Scorpion stings, 75
Sea salt, 125
　for bug bites, 37
　for poison ivy, oak, sumac, 74
　for radiation, 113
　for sprains and strains, 82
　for sunburn, 88
Seaweed
　for chemical contamination,
　　43
　for food, 109–10
　for radiation, 113
Second-degree burns, 39, 42
Seizures or convulsions,
　75–77. *See also* CPR
Severed body parts, 33
Shepherd's purse, 122
　for abrasions and lacera-
　　tions, 23
　after childbirth, 99, 100
　for nosebleed, 70
Shiitake mushrooms, for
　stress, 44
Shock, 77–78. *See also*
　Recovery position

Siberian ginseng, for heat
stroke, 65
Skullcap, 122
for burns, 42
for seizures or convulsions,
76
Slippery elm
for diarrhea, 47
for stomach pain, 87
for throats, irritated, 45
Snakebite, 78–80
Spider bites, 80–81
Spider webs, for abrasions and
lacerations, 23
Spinal injuries, 18, 29
Spirulina, for burns, 42
Splints and slings, 16–17, *17*
Spongia tosta, for asthma
wheezing, 28, 124
Sprains and strains, 81–83
St.-John's-wort, 121, 125
for burns, 41
for spider bites, 81
for sunburn, 89
Staphysagria, 124
for bug bites, 38
Stingray stings, 83–84
Stings (bee, hornet, wasp),
84–86. *See also* Jellyfish
stings; Scorpion stings;
Stingray stings
Stomach pain, 86–87. *See also*
Food poisoning; Vomiting
Strawberry, for diarrhea, 47
Stroke, 87–88. *See also* CPR
Sulphur, 124
for diarrhea, 48
for poison ivy, oak, sumac, 74
Sunburn, 88–89. *See also*
Burns; Heat stroke
Swedish bitters, for poison ivy,
oak, sumac, 74
Symphytum, for fractures to
face, 58, 124
Taurine, for seizures or con-
vulsions, 76
Tea bags, for burns, 41
Teas. *See* Black tea; Green tea
Teas, herbal, 128
Tea tree essential oil, 119
for abrasions and lacera-
tions, 23
for animal bites and
scratches, 26

for bug bites, 38
for burns, 40
for mosquito bites, 36
for sprains and strains, 82
for toothache, 90
Third-degree burns, 39, 40, 42
Ticks, disease from, 37
Tienchi ginseng, for abrasions
and lacerations, 23
Tinctures, herbal, 129–30
Toast, burnt, for poisoning, 72
Tobacco, for insect stings, 85
Tofu
for bruises, 35
for burns, 40
for sprains and strains, 82
Tomato leaves, for bug bites,
38
Toothache, 89–90
Tornado survival, 113–14
Tourniquet, 33
Trees for food, 110
Turmeric, 122
for sprains and strains, 83
Ume concentrate, 125
for diarrhea, 47
for food poisoning, 56
for stomach pain, 87
for vomiting, 92
Unconsciousness, 91. *See also*
CPR; Fainting; Head
injury; Recovery position
Urine
for jellyfish stings, 68
for poison ivy, oak, sumac, 74
Urtica urens, 124
for burns and stinging pain,
41
for sunburn, 89
Valerian, 122
for toothache, 90
Veratrum, 124
for bleeding and shock, 24
for heat stroke, 64
Vespa, for wasp stings, 85, 124
Vinegar and honey, for food
poisoning, 56
Vitamin A&D ointment, for
diaper rash, 45
Vitamin C, 125
for animal bites and
scratches, 26
for bruises, 36
for burns, 42

for food poisoning, 57
for frostbite, 60
for heat stroke, 65
for jellyfish stings, 68
for mosquito bites, 36
for nosebleed, 70
for snakebite, 80
for stings, insect, 86
Vitamin E, 125
for burns, 42
for frostbite, 60
for jellyfish stings, 68
for sprains and strains, 83
Vitamin K, for bruises, 36
Vomiting, 92
Watermelon, for heat stroke,
64
Water shortage survival,
114–16, *115*
Wheat germ oil, for burns, 42
Wheat grass, for bruises, 35
White oak, 122
for bug bites, 37
for diarrhea, 47
for poison ivy, oak, sumac, 73
Windpipe, preventing blockage of, 18, *18*
Witch hazel
for heat stroke, 64
for mosquito bites, 36
Wounds. *See* Abdominal
injuries; Abrasions and
lacerations; Bleeding
Yarrow, 122
for abrasions and lacera-
tions, 23
for fever, 55
for nosebleed, 70
Yeast, for diarrhea, 47
Yellow dock, 122
for nettle rash, 68
Yogurt
for burns, 41
for diaper rash, 45
for diarrhea, 47
for food poisoning, 57
for sunburn, 89
Zinc
for burns, 42
for frostbite, 60

OTHER STOREY TITLES YOU WILL ENJOY

Dandelion Medicine, by Brigitte Mars. This much-maligned weed is in truth one of the safest and most effective medicinal herbs available, with the power to fight infection, relieve congestion, aid digestion, and boost the immune system. Learn how to use this common plant in both food and home remedies. 128 pages. Paperback. ISBN 1-58017-207-5.

Healing with Herbs, by Penelope Ody. This visual introduction to the world of herbal medicine offers clear, illustrated instructions for growing, preparing, and administering healing herbs to relieve ailments such as arthritis, asthma, ear infections, is, depression, headaches, infertility, colds, fever, acne, eczema, allergies, and m re. 160 pages. Hardcover. ISBN 1-58017-144-3.

Herbal Antibiotics, by Stephen Harrod Buhner. This book presents all th ent information about antibiotic-resistant microbes and the herbs that are most ive in fighting them. Readers will also find detailed, step-by-step instructions for ing and using herbal infusions, tinctures, teas, and salves to treat various types o fec- tions. 144 pages. Paperback. ISBN 1-58017-148-6.

The Herbal Home Remedy Book, by Joyce A. Wardwell. Readers will discover how to use 25 common herbs to make simple herbal remedies. Native American legends and folklore are spread throughout the book. 176 pages. Paperback. 1-58017-016-1.

Rosemary Gladstar's Herbs for the Home Medicine Chest, by Rosemary Gladstar. Discover the healing properties of common herbs like calendula and comfrey, then learn how to transform them into medicinal teas, tinctures, salves, oils, and syrups. Readers will find first-aid treatments for problems like burns, cuts, rashes, headaches, and colds. 96 pages. Paperback. ISBN 1-58017-156-7.

Saw Palmetto for Men & Women, by David Winston. Respected herbalist Winston brings a new perspective to using this popular herb for both men's and women's health problems such as prostate enlargement, male baldness, ovarian pain and cysts, infertility, cystic acne, anorexia, and as a booster for the immune system. 128 pages. Paperback. ISBN 1-58017-206-7.

These books and other Storey Books are available at your bookstore, farm store, garden center, or directly from Storey Books, Schoolhouse Road, Pownal, Vermont 05261, or by calling 1-800-441-5700. Or visit our Web site at www.storey.com.